pieces *of* me

pieces *of* me

veronica neave

Hegemony Press
An Imprint of Cedar Fort, Inc.
Springville, Utah

The opinions and views expressed herein belong solely to the author and do not necessarily represent the opinions or views of Cedar Fort, Inc. Permission for the use of sources, graphics, and photos is also solely the responsibility of the author.

References to dollar amounts in the text are in Australian dollars.

ISBN 13: 978-1-59955-851-6

Published by Hegemony Press, an imprint of Cedar Fort, Inc.,
2373 W. 700 S., Springville, UT 84663
Distributed by Cedar Fort, Inc., www.cedarfort.com

First published in 2009 in Australia by Big Sky Publishing Pty Ltd.

LIBRARY OF CONGRESS CATALOGING-IN-PUBLICATION DATA

Neave, Veronica, author.
  Pieces of me / Veronica Neave.
    pages cm
  Originally published: Newport, N.S.W. : Big Sky Publishing, 2009.
  ISBN 978-1-59955-851-6
  1. Neave, Veronica--Health. 2. Breast--Cancer--Patients--Biography. 3.
Breast--Cancer--Genetic aspects. 4. Breast--Cancer--Prevention. I. Title.

  RC280.B8N42 2011
  616.99'4490092--dc23
  [B]

                              2011014662

Cover design by Megan Whittier
Cover design © 2011 by Lyle Mortimer
Edited and typeset by Kelley Konzak

Printed in the United States of America

10 9 8 7 6 5 4 3 2 1

Printed on acid-free paper

This book is dedicated to my great-grandmother Maude Hutchins, my grandmother Elsie Clitherow, and my mother, Claudette Neave.

I wear your genes with pride on the inside.

contents

acknowledgments

I would like to thank my two lovely sisters, Christine and Elisha, for sharing the ride; my brother Denny for forcing me to write this book; and my father, Colin, and brother John for allowing me to write of their pain. Thanks to Sharon and Diane for keeping me honest.

Thanks in the millions to Sam for changing my dressings and sharing the load and to my beautiful little guy, Kaspar, for helping me heal.

Finally to all my friends and family who heard me bang on about my boobs for an annoyingly long time. I promise now to stop.

prologue

. . . .

'm fine! I feel great. It went really well. I feel great!" I heard a female voice calling boisterously. "I feel really good," she kept protesting. "And look—isn't it wonderful?" she cried as she lifted her hospital gown to reveal the mass destruction that, only hours ago, was two healthy breasts. It would be a few hours yet before I realized that this deluded but cheery woman was, in fact, me.

The perpetrator of this glorious delusion was a beautiful anesthetist who wore bright red lipstick and fabulous jewelry and assuaged my fears moments before surgery with promises of unnatural highs. "I'm going to give you this drug that will make you feel great. It's a really nice one—one of my favorites."

"What about the self-administered morphine drip afterwards? Do you think I could have that?"

"Well, you could but . . ." My legal pusher tempted me with her wares. "I'm thinking of giving you three-hourly injections under the skin. The drip will take away the pain, sure, but with the injections under the skin, not only will you feel no pain but you'll also feel really great in your head, if you know what I mean." I'm not sure I did know what she meant, not being a drug user myself, but a hospital seemed like a safe enough environment to get off my face for once.

Well, off my face I was. I felt no pain. I felt no sense of reality whatsoever, and considering the actuality of my situation, this illusory state was the best place for me. God bless my anesthetist! God bless hospital drugs!

Only hours later when the unrelenting, excruciating, unfathomable pain kicked in was I forced to face the truth that I had just had a prophylactic bilateral subcutaneous mastectomy at thirty-nine years of age in the hope of escaping a deadly heirloom that had ravaged generations of women in my family.

My great-grandmother Maude Hutchins, my great-aunt Dolly Gleeson, and my grandmother Elsie Margaret Clitherow all died of breast cancer by the time they were fifty years old. My mother, Claudette Clitherow, developed breast cancer at forty-nine, and her sister, Margaret, a little later at age fifty-nine. I was given a window—a looking glass—that showed me a future I did not desire, so I changed it.

1

in *the* beginning

· ·

My mother, Claudette Clitherow, idolized her mother, Elsie. From what Mum tells me of Elsie, I can understand why. She was strong, stoic, charitable, and compassionate. I also idolize Elsie—vicariously though, because I never met her. Mum had only one sister, Margaret, who was three and a half years her senior. Justified or not, my mother always felt that Margaret was the favorite. So young Claudette grew up desperately yearning for her mother's attention. When Margaret became engaged, Mum secretly rejoiced because she thought after the wedding she would finally have Elsie all to herself.

In 1962, the year of Margaret's wedding, Elsie was diagnosed with breast cancer. She had a mastectomy in March, followed by radium, and when she came home from the hospital, Elsie worked around the clock making the wedding dress and bridesmaids' dresses for Margaret's November wedding. I am so in awe of the way women of yesteryear had the ability to sew whatever they required. Sure, it may have been borne of necessity, but it's a skill that I wish I had. This ability was passed on to my mother; she made her own wedding dress and all of her bridesmaids' dresses. Then when she had her own family, she was prolific in her output of school uniforms, formal dresses, ballet costumes, and the like.

The month after Margaret's wedding, Elsie's condition deteriorated. She went to the hospital, but when it became clear she would not recover, Mum's father wanted her brought home. Elsie's mother, Maude, had died at home, and they wanted Elsie to do the same.

My mother sat vigilant by Elsie's deathbed. The story that Mum tells is she had purchased a bunch of roses for Elsie when they brought her home from the hospital. She put them in two little hand-painted vases that had belonged to Maude and set them on her dressing table. When Mum bought the roses, they were just buds, but one particular rose began opening faster than all the others. My mother said to her auntie, "Mum won't live longer than that fullest rose." Three days later, Elsie died. Mum sat in the room with her, waiting for the undertakers, and noticed the rose was in full bloom. She left the room when they came to take Elsie away, and when she went back in, every single petal on that rose had fallen—it was literally a stem. I believe my Mum never really recovered from the missed opportunity of being close to her mother.

A few nights after Elsie's death, my mother, who was a chronic asthmatic, had an attack in her sleep. She was lying there, trying hard to breathe, when she felt someone touch her on the thigh. My mother rolled over and saw Elsie standing there in her pink dressing gown. Mum said to Elsie, "I'm all right," and Elsie walked away. This calmed my mum enough to fall asleep.

It was Christmas Eve when Elsie died, and, ever since, Christmas has been a bittersweet time for my mother. We all sense her sadness on this night. She was only seventeen at the time, studying to be a nurse, and she stayed on at her Bundaberg home to look after her father, grandfather, Great-Auntie Phyllis, and their neighbor, old Mr. Blackburn. Phyllis had been brain-damaged from birth and needed constant care, and Mr. Blackburn, who was eighty-nine, had been cared for by Elsie for ten years. My mother thus began a long life of selflessly caring for people—strangers as well as family.

My mother met my father a year later on a blind date. My father, Colin Neave, wasn't supposed to be her date, but his own date didn't show. He was turned on by Mum's record collection, and so fate lent a hand, spinning a thread of love and dedication that has lasted over forty years. They married quickly to prevent my father's two little sisters—Jacquie, age ten, and Linda, age eight—from going into care. Dad's father had been killed in a hit-and-run car accident, and six weeks later, his mother died of pneumonia. She was an alcoholic and had severe cirrhosis of the liver; the pneumonia was simply too much for her already struggling body.

So my mother and father had an instant family to care for when they were both just twenty years old, and over the next twelve years, they had five more ankle-biters of their own. We moved around a lot, and at times our home was a haven for a menagerie of people my mother felt obliged to rescue.

My father's sisters, Jacquie and Linda, lived with us off and on for many years. Linda married and then divorced, so she came back to live with us again. Jacquie had a child, my cousin Brooke, and was a single mother, so they both lived with us.

At one stage, Mum took in a young soldier called Davo, who had no family, and a homeless drunkard called Uncle Max. We also took in foster children: a teenager named Alana and two newborn babies, Annie and Jennifer. My mother also sponsored an entire family of Ethiopian refugees immigrating to Australia, so Kiros, Solomon, Rosa, and Mulikin appear in our family photos over a number of years.

Then there was Arti, a tiny Dutchman with a hump who had survived Auschwitz. Arti lived with our family for the best part of twenty years. They had employed Arti as a cook once when they worked in the restaurant business, and it was then that my mother realized he was alone in Australia. My parents eventually attached a trailer to their Gold Coast house to accommodate him. He had many obsessive compulsive disorders due to his time in the concentration camp, and when he declined into Alzheimer's, he was intensely rude and difficult. He had not a friend in the world except for my mother, so she cared for him until his death at eighty years of age.

Mum's charity work didn't stop there. Some people go in for extreme sports, Mum practices extreme charity. She has volunteered for a charity called Rosie's for two decades, mainly working on the streets feeding, clothing, and befriending the needy. Rosie's is a not-for-profit organization that provides outreach services to those marginalized in our community. She initiated a program for Rosie's volunteers to visit inmates in both male and female prisons. She even taught the prisoners line dancing at one point.

This opened our house up to a few friendly felons who Mum thought she could help once they were released. There was Carol, the bank robber who apparently at one stage in her life was the most wanted woman in Australia. Mum also helped another bank robber named Marie get her life back on track. Then there was Jimmy. My mother just knew he needed some loving support when he was released if he was ever going to make it. He lived with us for a while, eventually got a job, and now is married with a baby. He says none of this would be so if it weren't for my mother.

I have asked Mum where this compulsion to commit serious acts of compassion comes from, and there is no doubt in her mind that it was passed down from Great-Grandma Maude to Elsie down to Mum herself. Maude would pick up drunks off the street and feed them and give them a bed for the night. Elsie, too, cared for a number of people throughout her life who were not related to her. I would love to be able to say that I've inherited these charitable qualities, but no such luck; my sisters and I suffer the same selfishness that afflicts most generation X-ers.

My father was a regular soldier in the Australian army when he met and married my mother in 1965. Within nine months, my sister Christine was born. My mother was a very strict Catholic, but if you do the math, it's obvious there was a bit of hanky panky before the wedding. I came along eighteen months later, on 24 October 1967. My father was posted to Malaysia when Mum was pregnant with me, so I was born in Malacca. My mother was very much on her own in a foreign country with two tiny tots. She had no mother to help guide her through early motherhood, a situation I can't even begin to imagine. She gave birth to all five of her children naturally, without even a sniff of hospital drugs.

In Malaysia, we had nannies known as "Ah Mas" who helped Mum with the chores and children. It was the way things were done there at that time. I remember little of those years, but I do recall our Ah Mas's names: Ah Choo, Ah Wee, Ah Mow, and Ah Swan. I also remember a big water buffalo in the rice paddock at the rear of the house.

After two years in Malaysia, we returned to Australia, settling in Brisbane. Mum was pregnant again, and my father was sent to fight in Vietnam. It was 1970. He was Sergeant Colin Desmond Neave of the 8th Battalion of the Royal Australian Regiment. He was away for 366 days, during which time my brother Denny was born, named Colin Denny after my father. Mum stayed at home with three children under five as well as Dad's two sisters. Mum wrote to Dad every single day he was away, but more often two to three letters a day. Dad told me he received over 1,200 letters. He still has them in a box somewhere. I can't wait to one day get my hands on them for a bit of salacious reading.

My father came home a different man. Before he went to Vietnam, he didn't drink. In fact, one disturbing story he tells proves this to be true. When he arrived at camp on his first day in Vietnam, he ran into a friend of his, platoon commander Lieutenant Convrey of the 9th Battalion, whom my dad had trained only a few short months before. This officer asked my father to have a drink with him in the mess, and Dad obliged, although he wasn't keen because he was not much of a drinker. They had one drink and then left the mess. The officer then tried to convince Dad to come back to his tent to get drunk. My father refused, saying he was tired. They parted company, and a few short minutes later, that officer's tent was blown up with him inside. I always remember this story because, had Dad been the drinker he is today, he would have died on the first day of his tour of Vietnam.

When Dad came back from the war in 1971, he began his slow decline into alcoholism. He got out of the army six months later, and Mum and Dad bought a restaurant in Brisbane city called the Cork and Fork. I remember this time—I must have been five—because it was the only time in our lives up until then and forever after that we had a brass razoo. We had a biggish house in Brisbane, with a leather lounge suite and carpet on the floor. I had a Sleepmaker bed. We had a Valiant Charger, lunch money, and a bar in the living room. I think these material things stand out for me simply because for every other time in my childhood, my memories seem defined by degrees of poverty.

At this time, I had a best friend named Pamela, who was deaf. I learned to speak to her in sign language. One day, one of our neighbors had a television delivered, and Pamela and I hopped into the back of the truck. I told her in sign language, "When I say 'Go,' we'll jump out." The truck driver started the truck and drove off slowly, and then I yelled "GO!" and jumped. Well, Pamela didn't jump. She didn't hear me, and I watched her little face get smaller as the truck drove off down our street. This is where that memory ends, but she must have been returned before too long because I have other memories of her.

One night Mum and Dad picked us up from the baby-sitter's house after closing the restaurant, and we arrived home to find two fire trucks in our driveway. Our house was still standing, but my bedroom was all but cinders. It seems little Pamela had snuck into our house that night and was playing with matches in my room. Ah, the good old days when you could leave your front door unlocked and little kids were allowed to play with matches!

Mum became pregnant with my brother John in 1975, the year that she and Dad became bankrupt. All I remember is a big truck taking away all of our things. I definitely remember saying to Mum, "Why are they taking away my Sleepmaker?" It must have survived the fire. We ended up sleeping on the floor of a family friend's living room for a while. In fact, Mum gave birth to John while we were still in this homeless state. Then we really hit the skids.

We moved into a fourteen-foot trailer in a trailer park in Ipswich. Jacquie and Linda went to stay with their older sister Loraine till we had a little more space. I didn't really register that we were living in extreme poverty. I was only about eight years old, but looking back, it was pretty dire. Mum and Dad would show up at the meatworks every morning before dawn to try to get a day's work.

Our family eventually moved into a thirty-two-foot trailer, and it seemed palatial in comparison. We had the bombiest of all cars because my father was not allowed to own anything that cost more than about five hundred dollars. Life in the trailer park was a bit rough. I remember being pushed over by a girl called Panda and covered in rhinoceros beetles as a friendly joke. We played "Truth Dare Double Dare" in the coal mines, where a boy kissed me for the first time, and it felt yucky and wet. But kids are so resilient. We just adapted and made the most of it.

My mother must have been struggling; four kids, bankrupt, in a trailer park with an alcoholic husband—not quite living the dream. But she always made ends meet somehow, and we never seemed to go without much. Mum would always say, "God will provide," and he did. One day, a washing machine turned up at our trailer with a card on it but no name. Another time, when we couldn't afford a turkey for Christmas, there was a knock at the annex, and there stood a stranger bearing a turkey.

In 1977, Dad reenlisted. It seemed the only way out of the impoverishment his family was enduring. We moved back to Brisbane and lived in an army house. This is when my mum started collecting people. As well as Mum, Dad, Chrissy, me, Denny, and John, we had Jacquie, Linda, and Davo, the young displaced soldier. I have fond memories of this house. Jacquie and Linda worked at a pastry factory, and on Fridays they brought home a big box of the yummiest things for us all. There were custard tarts, cream buns, lamingtons, and chocolate éclairs, to name but a few. We used to have egg fights, and absolutely no one escaped one of my mother's raw egg shampoos—Mum was always the most aggressive food fighter. I remember running under the sprinkler in the backyard in our swimsuits. I remember walking to school, almost two miles, and seeing the gas station attendant writing the price of gasoline on a chalkboard each day; it was about eleven cents a liter. On the way home from school, I would stop and buy ten cents' worth of mixed lollies from the corner shop in a little white paper bag.

I had a healthy hatred of my big sister, Chrissy. We fought over everything. Looking back, I think I resented how difficult it was for my mother to look after Chrissy.

Chrissy was always nearly dying from her asthma; you can imagine how heartbreaking it must be for a mother to have a fragile child. I didn't understand Chrissy's pains and afflictions. I just added to them by being a proverbial pain in the butt. I did once actually stab her in the butt cheek with a barbeque fork because she wouldn't do the washing up. I can now appreciate that my sister found it hard to do the washing up because her skin was always red, raw, and bleeding from her eczema.

During this time, when I was about ten years old, I became rather religious. Mum had always taken us all to church every Sunday on pain of death. She sent us to private Catholic schools; who knows where she got the money. I'm at a loss when I wonder how she could have afforded the school fees. Although, come to think of it, she used to always take little bits of food off our plates or ask for a bite of our ice cream when we had them as a treat, which was really annoying. I would say, "Mum, don't! Get your own." But the thing is, she couldn't get her own; she was going without all that time so we didn't have to.

I started to ask Mum to take me to Mass each morning. She was so thrilled. I think my mother had fantasized about being a nun at one point in her life, and since this had not happened, the idea of one of her daughters joining a cloister was tantalizing. I did have passing notions of living at home with my mother until I joined the Sisters of Mercy or the Carmelites, it's true, but the real reason for the daily devotions was a young altar boy named Anthony. Oh, how I loved him with all my heart and soul, and oh, how I wanted to kiss him behind the chapel.

In 1977, Mum had little Elisha, the final addition to our family. Like Christine, Elisha was born with terrible asthma. Christine had been in and out of the hospital all her life, and my mother spent many hours each week giving her "physio" at home. She would lay Chrissy over her knees, tummy down, cup her hands, and bang her lungs until my sister expelled tons of phlegm. It seemed Elisha would suffer the same fate.

When Elisha (or Bang Bang Loo Loo Bell Strawberry Cake Face, as we called her) was a few weeks old, Mum took her to the hospital because she wasn't well. The doctors sent Mum home and told her not to worry, but Loo Loo seemed to get worse. Mum showed up at the hospital again, like a lioness, and said, "I am not leaving this hospital—my child is very sick, I know it." Well, she was right, as mothers often are, and before long Elisha was in intensive care and not likely to make it through the night. My mother called the priest and had him give Elisha her last rites. Then ever so slowly Loo Loo crept back to us.

There we were, the Neave family, complete, and in the safest of hands: my mother's.

becoming me

My mother, because she had the power to turn water into wine, gave us every opportunity when we were children to be the best we could be. From the age of five, I went to drama classes as well as ballet, judo, ballroom dancing, and Scottish dancing.

I was hopeless at ballet because I was born with pigeon toes. The photos of me as a baby show my feet completely turned in toward one another. It was thought that ballet would train my feet to turn out. Well, it did to some degree, but by about age eight I had "failed" my third exam. How could that ballet mistress fail a little person who is doing their darndest? The reason I failed is that my left foot was slightly pigeon-toed. Had she not seen how far I had come? I still can't forgive the old battle-ax, and I love my slightly turned-in left foot—it just wants to be friends with my right one.

The Scottish dancing was a slightly obscure choice on my mother's part, but I did the Fling, the Swords, and the Sailor's Hornpipe for a good eight years of my little life. Chrissy was a Scottish dancer too. She was much better at it than I was. We used to go to competitions, and she would always win loads of medals, and I would come third or get a special commendation. Mum made all of our costumes except for the tartan skirts, which were bought, and very expensive, at that. I was crowned Miss Scottish Dancing Queen for the Blue Bonnets Association in 1977. I still love hearing the bagpipes played; it takes me to an innocent place.

Dad was posted to Darwin in 1979, and then we moved to the Gold Coast in 1982. But wherever we were living, I continued the drama classes, right up until the end of my schooling. I'm not sure if I was born to be an actor or if my mother provided me with the tools and I just became very practiced at it. Whatever the wellspring, it was a natural progression for me to try out for drama school after Year 12.

There is a hideous event at the end of high school in Australia called "Schoolies Week." It's supposed to be a celebration, a rite of passage, for young adults. But it's really just an excuse for young people to drink their body weight in alcohol and unleash themselves on each other very publically. What a messy time it is. My friends and I rented an apartment in Surfers Paradise for a week with the thousands of other "schoolies," but I can't remember leaving my room. I didn't like the taste of alcohol, and I had no desire to be drunk—there was hardly any romance in that for me. More important, I also needed to prepare my audition to apply to various drama schools. I was never one to be seduced by peer pressure, nor did I give a hoot what anyone thought of me. I was quite confidently my own person. This was never more evident than when I took an Aboriginal man as my date to the Year 12 formal. I didn't think twice about it—he was so cool—but the looks and stares I got from those around me were surprising. The jaws that dropped the lowest were the nuns'.

I worked arduously on my audition piece and choreographed a dance solo to the overture of *Jesus Christ Superstar* right there in our schoolies' living room. What a dork! Thankfully the audition was a success. My examiners raised their eyebrows when I performed my dance piece. Surely, I thought, their facial expressions meant they were stunned by my genius. They were stunned, all right, I think by my unadulterated audacity. They offered me a place right there and then to the acting school at the University of Southern Queensland. It was a good school and had a great reputation. I phoned my mother immediately after the audition and told her I'd been accepted. She cried. It meant that I would be leaving home to go and live in Toowoomba. My father had been posted to Townsville in Far North Queensland, so I would be thousands of miles from my family.

My father had become a bit of a stranger to me. He was never violent and always fair and supportive; he was just absent in his soul. My mother loved him madly and "sat like patience on a monument" waiting for him to be restored to her. Alcohol was not allowed in the house, but my father would find ways to annihilate himself. Sometimes he would pick us kids up from school and then pull the car off the road, and we would sit in silence as he drank two tallies. We would never say anything. Sometimes he would go out to wash the car. It would take him hours, and when he finished, he would come in drunk. We would find beer bottles stashed throughout the garden or under beds. My mother attended Al-Anon, a support group for the families of alcoholics, and tried very hard to find a way to help him.

I felt a great deal of compassion for my dad, even from a young age. I remember at seven years old I would pray to God to help him because I knew he was sad. Why wouldn't he be? He'd watched his best friend, my godfather, get blown to bits right in front of him and had tried to piece his body back together. There were too many bloodcurdling moments for him. He had nightmares and terrible trouble with his skin from Agent Orange, yet he never spoke to anyone about these things. He hardly ever spoke at all. He kept it locked inside and seemed powerless as it ate away his being.

My sister Chrissy had grown into a "troubled teen." She was always running away and hanging with the wrong crowd. She'd left school early and become pregnant by the time she was sixteen. My mother was beside herself with trying to control her, but once Chrissy had her little boy, David, she began to blossom into the person who she wanted to be.

My brother Denny was the perfect child. He seemed to recover from the torture of being dressed only in girls' clothes for the first five years of his life by his two wicked sisters. We also told him from a young age that he was adopted; in the end I think he wished he had been. He was studious and very well behaved—the golden boy. Growing up poor had given me a very easygoing attitude to money. The "God will provide" motto had been tattooed onto my psyche, and I always knew I would have enough. Denny, on the other hand, adopted a Scarlett O'Hara quality with a determination to never go hungry again.

You could see in his eyes he was going to be emancipated from poverty as soon as was humanly possible.

The other two, John and Loo Loo, were still littlies. These two became inseparable. The older children— Denny, Christine, and I—moved from home when we were all around sixteen years old. John and Loo never really left the nest. As they grew up, Dad's alcoholism got much worse, and they bore the brunt of it. He became darker and less sociable. My mum always tells me that I never saw how hard it was for John and Loo, and I believe her. As my little brother John grew older, he inherited the same disease as my father, and it has destroyed his life. My little sister is not an alcoholic, but she has her own health concerns, having struggled with anorexia, anxiety, and self-esteem issues.

University was so exciting. The theater faculty reflected every sort of cliché attached to "arty" types. We wore crazy clothes, sang the lyrics of daggy musicals through the corridors, and were basically self-absorbed and annoying. I really flourished in the artistic environment.

I was an individualist, and as this was a prerequisite for my degree, I could roller-skate to uni in my pajamas with confidence. Three years went by quickly. We were all so poor as students, though I was used to it. In the 1980s, university was free for everyone, but in order to live, I had to work bar jobs on the weekend. The girl I lived with during university came from a very wealthy background; her family lived in a mansion and had at least seven cars. I found out, years later, that their wealth was procured via less-than-legal means, but at the time, we had the best furniture of anyone on campus. On our first day of university, my flatmate's father dropped us off in his gold Rolls Royce. I was a little embarrassed. Still, there were many nights of Vegemite pasta; I was as skinny as a stick.

Toowoomba was dubbed the city of flowers. It was very pretty and freezing cold. The town was inhabited by extremely conservative retirees. Every time we put on a show with a swear word in it, there was a community outcry. I loved the whole share house experience because it reminded me of home. There were endless parties that usually ended with me placating the police at the front door while wearing nothing but an aluminium bikini and swathed in cling wrap. I was always the loudest and the soberest. I didn't drink a drop of alcohol at uni; to me it did not mean happiness. I missed my mother very much, often calling her at two in the morning to ward off the creatures of the night. I worked very hard and did very well in my studies.

I flew home to Townsville during the holidays on the old Hercules jets, courtesy of the army. Around this time, my mum started having trouble with her heart. She rode to the doctor's on her push-bike and told him she'd been having pains in her chest. The doctor listened to her heart and said, "I'm going to send you to the hospital now. Is there someone I can call for you?" Mum said, "No, my husband has the car today, so I'll just ride my bike." The doctor replied, "I didn't mean is there someone I can call to give you a ride. You'll be going there in an ambulance."

When Mum got to the hospital, they gave her an ECG, and the machine went totally crazy. The nurse said, "I'll just have to get another machine because this one isn't working." The next machine behaved in the same erratic way, and they realized it was my mother's heart that was out of control, not the machine. The doctors couldn't believe that Mum had waited so long to present herself because for her heart to be in such a state meant she must have been in severe pain. Mum never complained, ever. They flew her to Ipswich Hospital to see a heart specialist. It turned out that my mother had a prolapsed mitral valve and required some pretty sinister drugs to keep her heart regulated. She could remain on the drugs for a few years but would eventually need surgery to fix or replace the valve.

After Dad's three years in Townsville, he decided to retire. It was 3 August 1986. He was forty-two years old and had served for twenty-two years by then. He told me later that he went in to sign his discharge papers on the day of his retirement, and they said to him that he was still a soldier until the hour of midnight. Mum was in the hospital for her heart, so Dad was home alone. He bought a bottle of Scotch and put his entire uniform on, including all his medals. He sat in the living room next to an alarm clock set for midnight. When the alarm went off, he walked out to the back fence, took off his medals, and one by one threw them as far as he could. He then stripped off his uniform, threw it as far as he could, and went to bed. Two days later, his medals were returned to him. Someone found them and took them to the army base, and the army sent them back to my dad.

In 1986, my family moved back to Darwin to live after Dad left the army. Mum had loved the heat and the lifestyle when we had lived there previously, and my sister Christine lived there too, with her son David and her husband. When I graduated from university, I went to

Darwin and worked three jobs until I had enough money to set myself up in Brisbane and start my career.

I got work straightaway as an understudy in Tom Stoppard's *Night and Day* for the Queensland Theatre Company. In those days, all shows had understudies; it was a great training ground for fledgling actors. There is no such thing as an understudy anymore; it is a luxury the theater can no longer afford. I simply turned up every day and watched another actress do all the work. I had a small role in the show as well. I was part of an illusionary trick in the play where the leading actress ducked behind a couch and I popped up, with my back to the audience, dressed as her. I dropped my robe and walked off the stage buck naked. A debut, you might say.

In 1988, at the age of twenty-one, I got my first main role in a beautiful play called *A Spring Song*. We were opening out of town and going on a regional tour before the season in Brisbane. In those days, we toured on an old bus. The cast and crew set off to Cunnamulla, about an eight-hour trip, to meet with the director and designer, who were driving in a separate car with a senior actress. They never arrived. They had a car accident, and the designer was killed instantly and the others went to the hospital. We were to open the following night. In the theater, there's a saying that "the show must go on." Well, it's true, but it's a stupid rule. They flew in a new actress, we went on, and it was almost as if nothing had happened. We were very depressed the whole tour. The theater rarely allows for the intervention of nature or human frailty. Strange, since that's what plays are usually about.

Next I was in Tennessee Williams's extraordinary play *The Glass Menagerie*, also for the Queensland Theatre

Company. I think that out of all my jobs, this show is held in the highest esteem in my heart. When theater really hits the right note and every element comes into play in perfect harmony, it is a magical experience for audience and actors alike. This show was enchanting. I can't think about it without getting goose bumps over my body, so visceral is the memory. Playing Laura was completely consuming. She was as fragile as a moth's wings and as innocently luminous as light through a crystal. I was given an enigmatic note from my director, Aubrey Mellor, to "act like a piece of glass." I thought, how can you act like a piece of glass? But that is what I did.

The next few years, I was in seventh heaven. I had the opportunity to play in numerous Shakespeare productions. I played Juliet, Viola, Cordelia, Bianca, Hermione, and Perdita. I also toured Shakespeare in schools for a few years. Performing Shakespeare is such a workout. The language is dense and rich, and the plays are emotionally epic and long. I consider actors to be athletes of the heart, and this is never more tested than when standing on the giant shoulders of William himself. There is nothing more glorious to me than speaking Shakespeare's words—well, perhaps there is one thing better, and that's speaking Shakespeare's words and being understood. How is it possible for one man to chronicle every possible degree of the human condition and do it with such clarity and beauty? Until the day I die I will be humbled by the gifts he has given me.

My mother would always come to see my shows. She would fly down from Darwin—either I would pay for it or she would pinch and save as she always did so mysteriously. I would not be surprised to learn one day that my mother moonlighted as a topless waitress or was the mistress of some oil baron—never for money but for food stamps, school fees, and diapers.

If it was a show in which I cried a lot or, heaven forbid, killed myself on stage, I would find her afterward in the toilets, unable to come out because her eyes were all puffy. She always said, "I feel like Elvis Presley's mother when she first saw him die in *Love Me Tender.*" Well, Mrs. Presley couldn't have gone through as many tissues as my mother has over the years; my mother has quite a big nose.

I was cast in an acting role in a show called *Body Slam* in 1992 with a contemporary circus company called Rock and Roll Circus. This changed the direction of my life. I was fascinated by the strength and rigorousness these people demonstrated. The human body is capable of such incredible feats, and I grew increasingly obsessed with putting my own body to the test. I began to train as an acrobat—as a hobby at first, but the more skilled I became, the more I could see that these disciplines would eventually make me a better performer. I grew muscles on my muscles; I started to look like a female body builder. I would carry huge men on my shoulders, hang by my toes on the trapeze, and stand on someone's head while they ran around the room. The stronger I got, the stronger I wanted to become. I trained for hours every day and went to the gym every morning before work to do conditioning. When I was touring Shakespeare to schools, the students would often ask why I had such big muscles, and I had the opportunity to say to all those young people that girls could be strong too!

This obsession with using my entire body as an

instrument for storytelling developed over the years, but initially the acrobatic path and the acting path never crossed. Only with dedication and careful manipulation did I eventually introduce the two crafts to each other, and they became friends.

3

a blot *on the*

. . . .

landscape

After about seven years of working in Brisbane, I moved to Sydney for the opportunity to work with other companies. It was 1993, and for the next decade I lived in "The Brighton Boulevard House." This house was about one hundred yards from Bondi Beach, and I shared it with a bunch of actors. I get very nostalgic for this period in my life, which was filled with so much joy and laughter, excitement and madness.

I thrived in the share house situation because it reminded me of the multitudes that were always at my home when I was growing up. The people in the Bondi house became my family. There was Paul (an actor), his fiancée, Elise (a painter), Christopher (another actor), Fleur (a singer), and Paula (an actress), each and every one uniquely talented and exquisitely insane.

Of course, we collected many other stray and

struggling artists through the years. At one point, there was a French painter/rock star living in the garage and another French photographer in a tent in the backyard. People were drawn to this house, and it became legendary for its all-embracing hospitality and guarantees of good times.

In my twenties, I was invincible. It's such a potent time—you're still free enough from cynicism to give people the benefit of the doubt. Free enough from responsibility to take risks. Free enough to not waste time worrying what consequences tomorrow may bring. Optimism outweighs fleeting concerns, and boundless energy prevails.

Don't get me wrong, I'm glad my twenties are over—it was exhausting. In my twenties, I could not sit for hours and meander through the tantalizing passages of a beautifully crafted novel. If I was reading a book, I was wasting time, being lazy. After yoga practice, you are meant to lie down in savasana (the corpse pose) for fifteen minutes of stillness that allows your mind to return home to you. In my twenties, I would sneak out of savasana because I couldn't bear to be still for more than a nanosecond. Now when I practice yoga, savasana is my reward.

One of the reasons I loved the Bondi house so much was that it was the first house I had lived in for more than two years in a row. My family had moved so much over the years, finally settling on the Gold Coast in 1990, that there is not one place that I would call my home. My home was just wherever my family was at any particular time. I think this constant moving has left me quite adaptable to new circumstances, but on the flipside, I can move on a little too efficiently, sometimes using detachment as a shield to ward off sorrow.

But I did become attached to the Brighton Boulevard house. It was also the most beautiful place on earth. The northern headlands at Bondi Beach are so stunning— the expressive sandstone cliffs, the balmy weather, and the blue Pacific Ocean with its enigmatic and humbling power. Every day I was there, I felt like I had paid a million dollars to be on vacation in the most dazzling of all destinations.

My career was moving along nicely. I did a few shows at the Sydney Theatre Company, had some small roles in feature films, and landed a lead role in a telemovie. My heady lifestyle, though, was interrupted by the specter of the cancer that claimed my great-grandmother Maude and my grandmother Elsie and that was now about to threaten my own mother.

It was 1995 when my mother was diagnosed with breast cancer after her very first mammogram. At this time, breast cancer awareness was increasing, but there were still heated debates about the cost-effectiveness of a national screening program. Breast conservation surgery was considered a better option than radical mastectomy because of the increased understanding of the psychological effects of removing women's breasts.

Funny enough, the year my mother received her diagnosis was the year that the BRCA2 gene (the breast cancer gene) was discovered by Professor Mike Stratton and Dr. Richard Wooster of the Institute of Cancer Research in the UK. Researchers have since discovered that mutations in the BRCA2 gene cause an increased risk of breast and ovarian cancer. Exactly ten years later, that little BRCA2 gene would turn up in Mum's blood test.

My mother didn't even bother to mention to the rest of her family that she had breast cancer. She just popped off to the hospital and had a lumpectomy. A few days later, her doctor called to say she needed to come in to have the whole breast removed, to which my mother answered, "Well, I'm a bit busy. Can it wait a little while?" He replied, "If you don't come in immediately, you will be dead by Christmas." With Christmas a mere five months away, she obeyed. We sort of noticed things were amiss when Mum came home less one entire breast.

The news then spread like wildfire through the family that Mum had cancer. To the public at large in the 1990s, cancer was still shrouded in mystery. The word still tended to mean certain death. My sister Christine remembers having a bad dream that she was at Mum's funeral, which she woke from in a state of hysteria. When she called home and discovered Mum had just had a mastectomy, Christine proceeded to scream down the phone at her for not telling anyone. The next day, she made arrangements to pack up her life in Darwin and move to the Gold Coast to be with Mum because, like the rest of us, she thought Mum must be dying.

My brother Denny remembers receiving a desperate call in the middle of that night from Christine. Although he doesn't ever recall crying in his adult life, he curled into the fetal position and sobbed. I must have received the call as well, although I don't remember it specifically. What I do remember is that it was the first time I had ever thought about death as more than an abstract idea. I remember being quite "together" about it, although I started having heart palpitations. Years later, I found a drawing I had done at that time that was horrifically telling. It was a charcoal sketch of Jesus Christ with one breast and a horrendous scar where the other one should have been. My mother had always been very religious, and I threw all of my anger at the God she had worked for and worshipped all her life.

As it turns out, Mum pulled through without a hitch and was back digging in the garden a week later. She did not require any radiation or chemotherapy. Mum just got on with it as usual and continued to protect the family from what she thought was unnecessary worry. Mum's desire not to worry us became pathological, and I began to find it terrifically frustrating.

One Christmas, a few years after her mastectomy, Dad let slip that she'd had a stroke and had failed to inform anyone. She tried to deny it, saying that Dad was just drunk. I really got mad this time. "Mum, please, you could be robbing us of the opportunity to say good-bye or to even help save your life." She just told me I was over-reacting. "It was nothing. I was just watering the garden and then I saw all these beautiful fairies flying around." Apparently she'd stood frozen in that watering position for about two hours.

I don't want you to get the picture that my mother is a sickly woman, although it seems she's had more than her share of health problems. If you met her, you would see she's very robust—as strong as an ox, in fact. She has this indefatigable might that I cannot fathom. There's something about the inherent strength of women from my family's past that seems to have diluted to a mere trickle over time. I just say their names—"Maude Hutchins," "Elsie Margaret Clitherow," "Claudette Clitherow"—and feel a wave of stoicism emanate from a bygone era.

For me, life went on, and I went back to concentrating on my career. Just as things were flowing on down the highway of success, I took a sharp exit stage left. In 1996 I was offered a job as a full-time member of a physical theater company aptly named Legs on the Wall. These guys were hard-core acrobats. Their shows were renowned for intense and somewhat dangerous physicality, and at this particular time, they were Australia's leading physical theater company. Legs on the Wall aimed to lend their intense physicality to narrative to tell more human stories than traditional circus or pure acrobatics. At the time, it was groundbreaking. They pushed these barriers further by offering me a position. They had never employed a trained actor before, but because my skills were high acrobatically, it seemed like quite a coup.

I was slightly terrified by my decision to join them. I would be moving away from mainstream acting and entering a world of rigorous daily training, crash mats, harnesses, sweat, sore muscles, calluses, and injury. What was I thinking? I embraced it with a certain suspension of disbelief and spent five years as a real-life acrobat.

It was an amazing job, really. We traveled the world. I had only been to Italy before on a vacation, but I got the chance to perform in Edinburgh, London, Brussels, all over Holland, and in British Columbia. Traveling with shows in this way is fantastic because you are not merely a tourist. You get to work with local people, and you really see the daily machinations of whatever city you are in.

Sometimes we'd perform our shows on the vertical face of a city skyscraper while we were suspended in harnesses. Looking back, I can't really believe it was me up there; I was actually afraid of heights to start with. It was extremely demanding work, and I could hardly get out of bed without the aid of an osteopath, but boy was I fit. I busted a disc in my back and injured just about every muscle known to man, but I survived, and I do look forward to telling my grandkids that old Grandma Ronnie was once a professional acrobat.

After five years, I grew a little weary of hurting my body so much. When I was working, I would use my body so vigorously that on weekends or holidays I'd be nursing injuries or trying to recuperate. It was all the wrong way around. I wanted to be more adventurous and vigorous in my life and less in my work.

As a young performer, your work is your life. When you're not performing, you're just waiting for the next time you will be. You are defined by your work. You are identified by the roles you have played, and you are only as good as your last performance. I know actors who, when they are not working, completely fall apart because they have no idea who they are or what to do with themselves outside trying to please an audience.

My achievements with Legs on the Wall were tangible. I could execute this particular trick, and I had mastered that particular move. I had proved that I could train and become an acrobat, and I didn't need to do it anymore because it hurt too much now. I had proved it to myself, not to anyone else. As actors, we are always trying to prove ourselves to others, and it is not healthy. It is because our performances are so ephemeral; once the show is over, it's gone, and there is nothing to prove that it happened—that magic happened. The audience carries the experience away in their heads and then forgets about it. So you end up chasing some proof of your existence: an old photo of when you played Juliet, a clipping of a review that said you were "as pervasive as a tantalising aroma." That's why many actors want to be film stars, perhaps.

In 2000, I began working for a company called Force Majeure. "Force majeure" is actually a legal term that means "superior force" or "act of God." I love this term because it can be used to defend oneself against all things inexplicable in life—quite handy, really. "Force" is a dance theater company incorporating movement and text to create original works that are quite spectacular. Kate Champion was the director, and I had worked with her once before.

This inspiring company was just where I wanted to be in contemporary Australian theater. Kate's goal was to fuse the language of dance and other forms of movement with text and spoken word. It is a hard thing to achieve. Usually people who are very skilled in dance or movement don't have confidence in speaking or acting, so the story can end up being too abstract, superficial, or lacking in emotional integrity.

But movement can be so incredibly expressive when exploring the human psyche, and words—well, words are fundamental in challenging our emotional intelligence. Imagine these two disciplines complementing one another fluidly when tackling important human stories. Kate was about to push against any confines and forge new ground in Australia. I was privileged and excited to be part of it.

Force Majeure's first show premiered at the Sydney Opera House for the Sydney International Festival in 2002. The show was called *Same, Same but Different* and was enthusiastically received. It set a new benchmark in storytelling for Australian theater. Kate and the Force company created *Same, Same* over ten weeks by improvising around specific themes, devising text and movement, and using large screen projections of material we had filmed. *Same, Same* won the award for most outstanding theater piece that year at the Helpmann Awards.

I went on to create two more shows with Force, which toured nationally and internationally. The last show, called *The Age I'm In*, won the most outstanding production for 2009 at the Australian Dance Awards. I love this work so much—it is still very physical but distills the best of both worlds of theater that I've been trying to straddle for so long.

4

life goes on

· ·

Four years after her breast cancer scare, my mother came with me on one of my tours overseas. She had hardly traveled out of Australia, mainly because she could never afford it, but she saved up her fare and came to England. Because all my accommodations were paid for, it was more affordable for her. After the tour, we traveled to Ireland together and then to Rome. At the time, she annoyed me, needing to pee every fifty yards and spending her precious little money on gifts for me and the family.

When we were in Rome, we went to the Vatican, and there was an enormous crowd. Mum said, "Maybe the Pope is here." I said, "Mum, don't be ridiculous. You can't just show up at the Vatican and expect to see the Pope; don't get your hopes up." But she was right: on that random day we went to the Vatican, the Pope happened to be there. It's every Catholic's dream, and it made her so happy.

She really is an adventurous person, and quite color-ful, with her hair dyed bright red. She'll do anything, talk to anyone, and go anywhere just for the experience.

She is quite mad, though. On the plane home, she was complaining about "Knoxy." I asked, "Who is Knoxy?" and she told me he was a little ghost she picked up in Exeter that wanted a free ride to Australia to see a cousin of his. When we'd been back in Australia a few weeks, she was still cursing "Knoxy," who, she says, was causing havoc all over the house. Apparently he soon hitched a ride back to England and never bothered her again.

One thing I noticed when we were away was that she missed my dad. I could tell she was pining for him even though before we left she couldn't wait to get away from him. He had been diagnosed as TPI (Terminally and Permanently Incapacitated) and stayed at home 24/7 watching his Westerns and drinking. My mother was such an energetic person with a voracious appetite for life, so it was sad to see her stuck at home with dwindling hopes that Dad would ever again share her happiness. She had given up banning alcohol in the house and had tried to leave him a number of times, but they were inextricably linked and probably always will be.

My brother John, too, was a full-blown alcoholic by the time he was thirty. He was very depressed and moving further away from the lovely, sensitive young man that he used to be. He had been to rehab a few times but relapsed each time. Is it in the genes? My father became an alcoholic; my father's mother was an alcoholic. Or was it because of John's upbringing and environment? We were all exposed to Dad's alcoholism though, and only John seemed to have suffered this misfortune. I yearn to have my little brother back—he suffers so terribly.

At home, Arti, the Holocaust survivor, was also

becoming more and more confused by his Alzheimer's and seemed to take out all his frustration on his primary caregiver, who was Mum. When I was visiting my parents from Sydney, I would see him be so rude to her at times, and then he would slip me five bucks and whisper, "Go get your mother something nice, darlink." Mum had a lot to cope with, but the harder things got at home, the more time she spent out of the house doing charity work.

My little sister Loo Loo (Elisha) was all grown up and in 2002 had her beautiful baby, Jack. Jack's father's name is Joe. Elisha and Joe met in Paris at World Youth Day in 1997. She was nineteen, and he was eighteen, and they decided then and there that they were going to be in love with each other for their whole lives and, to varying degrees, so far they have been. They have come close to getting married many times but keep canceling—well, to be fair, Elisha keeps canceling. They have also broken up that many times—well, to be fair, again, it is Elisha who has broken up with Joe. It seems she can't live with him or without him.

Denny went to university and studied business, of course. Mum always knew she would never have to worry about him. He had emulated Michael J. Fox's character in Family Ties down to a T, got a great job, and started making good money right away. He found his soul mate, Sharon, at university, and they seem to keep each other honest.

Christine divorced her first husband. They'd married far too young and for the wrong reasons. She met and fell in love with Ray, and they have been together now for about fifteen years. Chrissy developed a love for a style of partner dancing known as the Lindy Hop; it is a dance done to swing music. Ray just happened to be the greatest of Lindy Hoppers, and together they were simply astonishing. They won so many competitions that there was a demand for them to open a school for Lindy Hop, so "Katz Korner" was born. Ray is a man of the land by day, and Chrissy is a PA to an entrepreneur, but by night they don their fifties outfits and dance like there's no tomorrow.

I'd had numerous love affairs over the years. I guess I was a serial monogamist. Every time I began a relationship, I believed it to be the love of my life, and I was 100 percent committed. I was very affectionate, demonstratively so, and was always all-consumed with my lover of the moment. I was good at relationships, I think, and I was good at letting them go when I felt they'd reached a natural conclusion.

In 1998, as I was nursing a broken heart, my housemate Paul, aka Cupid, invited Tobias to our house for dinner. What can I say? Within six months we had decided to marry. I had wanted to marry just about every man that I went out with at one stage or another, but Tobias was it. He was tall and handsome, he was completing his doctorate in defense strategy, and he was smart. I would never need to worry about money, and he totally adored me. Toby was very black and white; once he made his mind up about something, it was absolute, and he had made his mind up about me. Before he'd even met me, he saw me from a distance and said to a friend, "I am going to marry that girl." And so he did.

I can't remember feeling that Toby was my soul mate or anything like that, but it was just absolutely the right thing that we should marry. I felt with such certainty that Tobias would adore me always, be loyal to me always, protect me always. He had a glorious smile and a masculine energy. If Tobias heard a scream in the night, he would jump out of bed and run into the night chasing the bad guy. He really did this on many occasions. It freaked me out. It's not that he was violent—he had never been in a fight, ever—but he had an unusual bravery mixed with a sense of righteousness.

What a beautiful day the wedding was. My family was there, my Brighton Boulevard family was there—it was just a blur of perfection. We married at the Sydney Theatre Company Wharf, right on the harbor underneath the bridge. Million-dollar views and Tobias, six foot two, in Armani, telling me "not to be afraid."

I'm not sure why it was that a year later I pulled the pin on the marriage. There was nothing wrong with our relationship. I think I was scared, which is such a generic excuse, but I don't know what else to say; it remains a mystery even to me. We had decided to marry after knowing each other for only six months. I worried that I had no idea who Tobias was, and now I was bound to him for all eternity. So instead of staying—to get to know him in earnest—I walked away, with all the coldness of a wet fish. I think I broke his heart. I know I broke mine.

My next relationship was with Nathan. If Tobias was a knight in shining armor riding a white steed, then Nathan was Tom Waits bareback on a brumby. Nathan was devilishly handsome and the funniest person I'd ever known. He was a wild spirit who blew into my life, untamed, untamable. I laughed for four years straight. When we met, I was in my early thirties, and after four years, that ubiquitous biological clock began ticking right on cue. I had trouble imagining Nathan as a father to my children; he was not ready at that stage—he was still a child himself. I knew that if I stayed with him, I would probably miss my opportunity to be a mother. He wouldn't be ready for years, and my eggs weren't getting any younger. I know that when the time comes, though, he will be a special father.

When we separated, I didn't think it was probable for me to meet someone, get to know him, fall in love, and decide to have children together all within a few years. I was almost thirty-five and knew the possibilities for having defects in my eggs were growing exponentially. I was definitely not looking for someone to have a baby with; I just figured being single was a good start.

5

motherhood

· ·

On 18 August 2003, Kaspar was born. I was thirty-five years old. I had been single only a few months when I met Sam, Kaspar's father. We had no plans to have a baby at all—we barely knew each other—but within a split second, I was pregnant.

Sam and I met while working on a show together. Sam was quite a bit younger than me—fifteen years, to be exact. He was pursuing me with all the effervescence of youth, and he was irresistible. I did try to forbear, though, as his age was a real stumbling block to me. But his youthful insistence wore me down, and we entered into a crazy affair for a few months. Although he was an amazing person, and gorgeous to boot, I didn't see us having any future together because of his age. He was just about to explode into the person he dreamt of being, make thousands of discoveries, mistakes, and detours, and I was ready to read long novels by a cosy fire. I explained this to him only a week before I started to pee at five-minute intervals. It was a very difficult situation because, although I was at a point in my life where I was ready to be a mother, how was it possible that Sam, given his age, was ready to be a dad? He was twenty, and I was devastated that he was now in this predicament.

I told Sam unequivocally that I was prepared to be, and more than capable of being, a single mother, but if you knew Sam, you'd know that this was never going to happen. Although young in age, he is much evolved in spirit. He was in shock at first, but he was determined to be the best father he could possibly be—and he is.

I packed up my Bondi belongings and headed north. This was much harder to do than I anticipated. I loved that house, I loved my family there, and I loved the life that it had given me. Bondi was the perfect place for me to be as a young, single, career woman, but it would not accommodate me as a mother. Sydney is too expensive, and being pregnant, I would not be able to work for long in my industry. I also felt I needed to be close to my family for this new chapter of my life.

I grieved for my Bondi life for a long while. It was hard to leave all my still-childless buddies. I felt like I was leaving the coolest party in the world unfashionably early and stone-cold sober. It was the first time in my life that I actually missed somewhere; I didn't think it was possible to be that happy again. I thought that that was it—I'd had my time in the sun. How wrong I was.

Although extricating myself from the Bondi clan was painful, I was more than ready to embrace the life that awaited me: being a new mother and living who knows where with a young man I barely knew. Like I said, I had always been good at adapting to new situations. I loved being pregnant so much. I was fortunate enough to have an easy pregnancy. I swam three days a week, practiced yoga right up until the birth, and felt just radiantly fantastic. I marveled at the changes in my body. My bum got so fat. I was getting changed one day in front of Elisha, and she burst out laughing. "What?" I asked. "I have never seen you with a fat bum before." She guffawed, rolling about and pointing at my bottom. I looked in the mirror. My bum was about twice its normal size and full of cottage cheese–like dimples. My breasts were huge— they had never been much bigger than a teacup, but they were now full of fecundity.

I set up house with Elisha, her partner Joe, and baby Jack on the Gold Coast. Sam was still living at his parents' house but spent much of his time with us. I hadn't lived in the same city with my family, let alone the same house as any of them, since I was sixteen years old, and it was a bit of a culture shock. When you live with a bunch of people to whom you are not related there is respect for personal space, and some basic courtesies are practiced. With family, there's an abrupt shorthand when it comes to your feelings and no such thing as politeness or unnecessary kindness. This offers a certain truthfulness, I guess, but taking people for granted just because they are your family is just laziness, and I fell into it like a slovenly pig as much as those around me did.

Being around my family also brought home the reality of Dad's alcoholism. Of course, I had seen snippets of it over the years when I visited, but being around it on a daily basis was sobering. I understood the degree of difficulty that my mother faced. On the phone, she was always complaining about Dad's drinking, but when I saw him on holidays, he was the "happy" drunk that we had grown to love: a good storyteller, a bit of a larrikin. But there is no such thing as a happy alcoholic. There are symptoms such as sleep apnea, liver failure, and black moods. And for family, there is the daily reminder that the person you love is slowly and methodically committing suicide right in front of you.

My brother John was on a bungee cord between hope and despair. He really wanted to stop drinking—I saw it in his eyes. I imagined him looking around and thinking, "Why is everyone around me allowed to enjoy life? Why have they all been awarded the opportunity to live and be happy, and I have not?" I wished I could help him. I would try and fail and give up, and then try and fail and give up again. It had been so easy to romanticize my family when I was in beautiful Brighton Boulevard. I could revel in the good times and just stick my head in the warm Bondi sand when it came to the messy stuff.

Living with baby Jack, however, was a joy and like boot camp for impending motherhood. He was a great kid, and I loved to be around him while I was growing one of my very own. I hadn't really spent a great deal of time with Elisha before; she was only six when I moved from home, and I was only now getting to know her. She had grown into a beautiful woman, striking to look at. When you went out with her, people's heads literally turned. I'm sure some blokes did themselves a neck injury. She was a curious mix of gregariousness and crippling self-doubt. And funny. I had always thought I was funny; it was my thing to be the biggest idiot in the room. But she was funnier, and she didn't even have to wear a red nose. Her humor was sharp, witty, and intellectually obscure.

Elisha suffered from postnatal depression, and as

smart and educated as we all thought we were, nobody even noticed till she had to ask for help when Jack was around twelve months old. It did initially affect her bonding with Jack, but slowly she blossomed into the mother that she knew she could be.

At about three months pregnant, I returned to Sydney to direct a show at the National Institute of Dramatic Art. My ultrasound showed a healthy, kicking baby doing what I am convinced was an advanced yoga pose. I was staying at the Bondi house while directing the show, and it was already starting to feel like I had moved on. The baby growing inside of me was like a beacon of light that threw anything behind it into shadow.

When I returned to Queensland, Sam and I set up house in preparation for the arrival of our new guest. We had a little apartment by the ocean on the Gold Coast. I tried to find a job, but it's amazing how it freaks people out when you turn up to job interviews with an enormous belly preceding you. I even went to an audition, and the director kept his eyes closed because the character I was auditioning for was not pregnant. I didn't get the job. I didn't get any work. I'd barely had a job other than acting in the last seventeen years; I felt like I could adapt to anything if I tried, but my "condition" seemed to betray me.

So I nested and gestated with all the enthusiasm and terror of a first-time mom. I also helped Mum with her charity work, visiting inmates in prison and teaching them line dancing. I went to the courts with her, where she handed out cups of tea and biscuits to people who were in serious trouble. She was amazing, never once asking anyone what their crime was; just listening and offering a nonjudgmental heart.

My water broke about an hour after I had a game of lawn bowls with Sam and his family. The excitement was greater than anything I had ever felt in my life. Curiously, the first person I called was my old partner, Nathan. He was so happy for me, and I knew he would be thinking of me during the labor, sending me his love.

The labor was, as many before have protested, so painful! I went for fifteen hours before screaming for the drugs. My mother was sitting there crocheting a baby blanket, never really looking up, just silently offering her presence. My sister Elisha was there too, curled up on a big chair and hungover from the night before. She was asleep for most of the labor except when I screamed too loud and woke her, and she would complain, "Give her the drugs." Oh, it's so easy for those who have already pushed a whole human being out of a ridiculously small hole.

Sam was beside himself trying to make me comfortable. He endured many fingernail wounds to his back as I hung onto him and moaned as if I was dying. When the doctor came in and said I needed to have an emergency Cesarean, I cried because I so wanted to have the baby naturally, and Sam cried, I think, because he thought this meant I was going to die.

In the operating room, I could see Sam was now freaking out. I tried to reassure him that everything would be fine and made him promise that he would not look at the surgeon taking out my intestines and laying them on my stomach. Somehow I knew this would not be a good look.

Kaspar was delivered, and in the delirium, I heard myself say, "Oh, thank goodness he doesn't have Down syndrome!" Sam was so proud, so happy, and so natural with his beautiful baby son. I had those amazing happy hormones buzzing around that counteract the shock that your body has just experienced. And so we began a love affair with our son that was, for both of us, the greatest love of all.

The next few months felt like I was covered in a cosy blanket and wandering through a misty maze of love and admiration. My nipples bled, I got mastitis (which is like someone fire-branding your already sensitive breasts), and I never slept more than one hour at a time for seven months. But these irritations would evaporate with an exhale as my eyes rested on a being that somehow brought clarity to the mysteries of my life. It seems that before Kaspar, I merely existed; now I was living.

When Kaspar was five months old, Sam and I took him with us to Sydney so I could help Kate develop a new show for Force Majeure. I had a freezer full of expressed milk for Sam to feed Kaspar after I left for work. At lunch I would empty my breasts while hoeing into a sandwich, and in the afternoon, Sam would bring Kaspar in for his midafternoon feed. Then I would race out the door at 5:30 p.m. to be home in time for the 6:00 p.m. feed.

My breasts were so full of the good stuff. I loved them. I was mesmerized by these mammaries that made milk to grow my son. The feeding itself was so beautiful that it would make me cry.

Once, at work, I was involved in an improvisation where I was hysterically crying and someone was doing everything physically possible to cheer me up. It was right at the end of the day, and usually you keep going in an improvisation until Kate calls stop. Well, the improv just kept going and going and no one was calling stop. The clock ticked past 6 p.m.—Kaspar's feed time—and my breasts just started gushing with milk. Tears were streaming down my face from the acting, and breast milk was streaming down my shirt. I just stopped and said, "I gotta go!"

Although everything was perfect with our son, I was deeply troubled by my feelings toward Sam. He was a great dad and a wonderful person, but I was not in love with him. I knew this before I became pregnant, but the news of the pregnancy and Sam's strong desire for us to be a family made me pull my head in and ignore my feelings. I tried very hard for about two years to fall in love with Sam. It would be perfect if I could: we had a beautiful child, he was the perfect dad, he was young and good-looking, and he was a really good person. Waiting for the but . . . but I did not love Sam in the way that I was pretending to, nor in the way he wanted me to. I loved him being the father of my child and I loved him as a companion and friend, but my intimacies with Sam were fraudulent. I discovered that you cannot make yourself fall in love with someone, just as you can never make someone fall in love with you. I wanted to, I really did, but love arrives only mysteriously, not on command.

It was the hardest thing I've had to admit to so far in my life. It was hard enough just to admit it to myself and own it, but then to have to admit it to Sam. I mean, it's one thing telling someone that you do not love them anymore, but to tell them that you never did in the first place! But I did it.

When Kaspar was two, the three of us moved to a five-acre property in a beautiful place called Tamborine Mountain in the Gold Coast hinterland. Sam and I bought the house with the assistance of my brother Denny. We are surrounded by hundreds of tall gum trees. There are kangaroos, koalas, goannas, and very deadly snakes. It is incredibly peaceful, and there is nothing to see but nature. If it wasn't so satisfying to absorb the serenity, I could feel very isolated, and sometimes I do. It's the opposite of the Bondi house yet equally special.

Kaspar and I live in the main house, and we built an amazing little place for Sam about one hundred yards away. We worked very hard to build a relationship that allows us to be a family unit, good parents, and good friends. It's worked. All of Kaspar's drawings show scenes of our cute little house plus Daddy's house plus Mummy and Daddy and Rusty the dog together. Sam has had a number of relationships with some beautiful ladies, whom I've welcomed with open arms. Kaspar is unaware of this part of Sam's life, but the arrangement is working for us so far. Most people around us said it would never work, but we expected that. Why not? Is it better to decide to hate each other and move very far away from each other and make the children pay for our selfishness? Sam and I actually really like each other, and I have never listened to what others say, anyway.

Although Sam has ventured into a few relationships, I haven't as yet. I felt guilty about hurting Sam by not being able to love him the way he wanted me to. It took me a long time to exorcise that guilt. The main reason, though, is that Kaspar has taken up my whole heart and there doesn't appear to be room in there for anyone else. If the right person came along, I'm sure that I'd quite easily and happily grow more heart to accommodate him.

Looking back, I'm lucky, really, that I did not have the complication of someone else in my life at this juncture.

The fates had other plans for me that all those except family would probably find too horrendous to deal with. The next chapter of my life would involve my dead ancestors, my mother's genes, and my two sisters and me making decisions in the present from projected outcomes in relation to the past that would ultimately affect our very existence in the future and include the removal of various body parts.

6

in my genes

Because of my family history, needless to say, when I was growing up there was a shadow of awareness that breast cancer was "in my genes." My great-grandmother Maude Hutchins died from breast cancer in 1925. She was born in 1875, only shortly before the first radical mastectomy was performed in 1882. William Halsted, an American surgeon, believed that removing the tumor and its "spreading tentacles" could cure breast cancer. These first radical mastectomies involved removing the affected breast, the nearby lymph nodes, and the two chest wall muscles. Maude died shortly after having her mastectomy.

By the time my grandmother Elsie Clitherow died of breast cancer in 1962, there had been developments in the treatments using radium and chemotherapy but also more extreme super-radical mastectomies that involved splitting the patient's clavicle, ribs, and sternum and then removing any organs and limbs thought to contain cancer. Irrespective of the "advances" in treatments, both my gran and great-gran died rather quickly after the discovery of their cancer. Elsie was treated with radium, which only seemed to make her last few months of life very difficult.

I never met my grandmother or great-grandmother, but from what my mother has told me, they calmly just accepted their diagnosis. The diagnosis in those days carried with it a strong likelihood of death. I find it fascinating imagining how the women in each generation of my family would have dealt with the news of their breast cancer. My mother says her mother was saddened at the thought that she would possibly soon be dead and that she'd never learned to play the piano properly. In Mum's eyes, her mother played the piano beautifully. In spite of it all, Grandma Elsie stayed positive and strong for the short ten months between diagnosis and death.

I didn't think too much about this skeleton in the closet during my invincible youth. However, it came to the forefront one day in 1999 when I was visiting my local GP in Bondi for a regular pap smear. Dr. Beth was an amazing doctor; it seems doctors like her just don't exist anymore. When you go to the doctor now, you've got only a few minutes, and too bad if you have several things to be checked out. Dr. Beth was always running late because she took as much time as was needed with each patient. You never minded waiting because you knew she would give you her most thorough attention. She was studying my records and, recognizing a pattern, suggested I visit a genetic cancer clinic at the Prince of Wales Hospital in Sydney. Even then, I went along not because I entertained the notion that I would ever get breast cancer but because I thought my curious heritage would help researchers know more about the disease. The research team seemed interested enough, so I signed up to help them—or so I thought. Over the next few years, I occasionally gave blood and filled out surveys about my health and psychological disposition.

Even when the clinic sent me a letter in 2005 asking if they could test my mother for a particular gene related to breast cancer, I remained blissfully unaware. "Come on, Mum," I cheered. "Help them save other women from breast cancer." When they located the BRCA2 gene in my mother in 2005, we were all a little clueless as to what that implied. She'd had cancer, and they found a cancer gene—seemed logical enough. They asked if they could test me to see if she had passed it on, and I was happy to comply. "Sure, if it helps science." I gave no thought to any possible outcomes from the test.

Now, I'm not usually one to stick my head in the sand or wade in denial, but I truly thought that I would never actually get breast cancer even though it was prevalent in my ancestry. I always felt as though I was different from the rest of my family. To start with, I was significantly different from my sisters. Christine and Elisha are both pretty and blonde, they both look more like my dad but inherited all of my mother's ailments, and they both have asthma and hay fever. In fact, the entire family has hay fever except for me. But I had failed to notice that I was the spitting image of my mother.

I took the test willingly, easily, and without a moment's thought and then promptly forgot all about it for six months. My mother had to remind me to obtain the results, and I made a rather blasé phone call to the clinic in early 2006. I had fallen through the loop, and they had forgotten to call me. The lady on the phone was a little confused and accidentally gave me the results then and there. I believe this is not normal protocol, but when she inadvertently confirmed I had inherited the mutation of the BRCA2 gene, I think I laughed out loud. I was obviously in shock, because I felt strangely elated, which seemed so inappropriate. I called all my family members to spread the astonishing news that I, Veronica, the one who was so different from all the others, had inherited a deadly heirloom passed down through all the women in my lineage.

I had no idea whatsoever what this result actually meant; this whole gene identification thing was so new we had never heard of it. I was not scared because I didn't know yet if it meant I would get cancer or that I was just a carrier; it was a mysterious bit of information to be holding.

In 2006, the Genetic Cancer Clinic sent me a letter of confirmation and arranged for me to see a counselor to talk through what all of this meant. The counselor gently explained to me what the BRCA2 gene actually was. BR is for breast, CA is for cancer, and the 2 means it is the second gene for breast cancer that was discovered. It was a bit of an out-of-body experience for me sitting there. I began to get the feeling that she was speaking to me as someone who was likely to get breast cancer. My brain tried to reject this information. How did I get here? And didn't this woman know that even though I had this so-called cancer gene, I wasn't really going to get breast cancer? I thought to myself that her sincerity must be helpful for people hearing devastating news but that it was wasted on me.

Kaspar was in the room with me, playing on the floor

with some toys. I just watched him while the counselor's dulcet tones lulled me into a pleasant trance. All I heard was, "blah blah blah breast cancer, blah blah blah breast cancer." I was thinking, "This can't be real." But there she was, looking at me intently, brandishing pamphlets and statistics.

Somehow I managed to come back into my body. The counselor continued her explanation in mellifluous tones, and I tried hard to focus on what she was actually saying. Apparently we inherit two copies of every gene: one copy from our father and one from our mother. Our parents, in turn, have inherited two copies of every gene from their father and mother. If one of your parents has a gene mutation in one of their copies, then they could pass on either the faulty copy or the correct copy to you, giving you a 50 percent chance of inheriting a faulty gene. Your genes provide the information for the growth, development, and function of your body. Genes are in every single cell, and in different tissues, they'll manifest in different ways. In your breast, the BRCA gene is what's known as a tumor suppressor gene. Its job is to keep the cells healthy and repair any possible abnormalities in the DNA. If you've got a mutation in your gene, it means there's a high risk that you'll develop an abnormality in a cell that will allow uncontrolled cell growth, which may turn into a cancer. Therefore BRCA2 mutation causes a predisposition to breast cancer.

In individuals with BRCA2 mutations, there is a significantly elevated risk of breast cancer—up to an 80 percent lifetime risk—and ovarian cancer, with up to a 60 percent lifetime risk ("lifetime risk" means the risk of developing or dying from a disease in your lifetime). The counselor began to map out my options and passed me all the available written information.

I sat on this information for many months until I finally understood and accepted that I was more than likely going to get breast cancer in the next ten years. It was a strange predicament because I wasn't told I actually had cancer, so there was no call for histrionics, but the warning of a ticking time bomb was not to be ignored. What emotional response was appropriate in this situation? I wasn't sure. I just felt weird, like I had overheard something I shouldn't have and didn't know what to do with the information.

7

keeping it
in the family

Following my cue, my eldest sister Christine decided to have the genetic test. I think it was more out of curiosity than any real fear. Because we have all been aware of breast cancer in our family for so long, there was almost a kind of complacency about it—if it's possible to be complacent about a disease that kills around 1.3 million women annually worldwide.

So off she went to be tested. Because I returned a positive result, I thought perhaps Chrissy wouldn't—we are so different. Or maybe I just hoped she wouldn't because she had already been dealt a bum hand with regards to her health. Her chronic asthma meant she had spent much of her childhood in hospitals. The drugs she had to take to treat her asthma made her teeth go very grey. She also had chronic eczema and was teased continually as a child about her rough and bloodied skin, even by me, I'm ashamed to say. However, in spite of it all, she grew into a beautiful woman. Enough already; let me be the one with the BRCA2 and finally balance out the inequity.

Her results took six weeks, and I think she was becoming quite anxious after learning what I now knew. Chrissy returned a positive result. She was not surprised. All of a sudden I felt closer to her than ever. Now we had each other to support—safety in numbers, sisters in arms. However, there was one more sister to go: our little sister, Elisha. She's the baby, she's the most beautiful, and she has always been the most vulnerable. Although Elisha is something of a stunner, she has struggled all her life with low self-esteem. This lack of confidence led her to get breast implants, which, in a superficial world, made her even more of a head-turner. We thought it would be a real blessing for her to be the one not to have BRCA2 to safeguard her already delicate physical confidence. We were all fairly certain that the odds would fall in her favor.

There is a 50 percent chance that any of Mum's children would inherit the gene mutation, and two out of her three daughters had already tested positive. Elisha put off the test for a long time. She joked that she wanted to be one of the gang, the "middle-aged mutant ninja chicks." But really, who in their right mind would want to be part of this posse? It took her about three months after Chrissy to decide to have the test. She tested positive.

I think my mother took this as quite a blow. She quite rightly felt no guilt about passing the gene on—how could she when it was passed on to her?—but to have all three of her daughters now in real danger of going through what she'd been through was a shock. We also have two brothers who could have it. There's a small risk of breast cancer in men who have the BRCA2 gene, and a slightly elevated risk of prostate cancer, but it's nowhere near as alarming as the risks for women. One of my brothers has a little girl, and should he test positive, there will then be a 50 percent chance that his daughter also will inherit the gene, and so on it goes.

Three sisters under forty years of age. I like to think of us as the "three graces": Charm, Beauty, and Creativity. Chrissy is a very good personal assistant to an entrepreneur and has her 1950s Charm School for Girls on the side. Elisha has a disarming beauty, some of which did cost her a fortune, but most of which she got from nature. I am the creative one, unromantically living on the bread line for the sake of art. Three sisters under the age of forty, armed with the knowledge that breast cancer was no longer a skeleton in the closet but a big fat elephant sitting on our laps.

How synchronistic that around this time, my mother found another lump at the site of the breast that a decade ago she'd had removed. We all reeled with a new sense of dread. This wasn't such a fun gang; it was a potentially deadly gang, and I was getting a little bit angry now at this ravenous and narcissistic gene robbing the world of strong and beautiful women. I never got to meet my grandmother who died in such pain, and I was not ready to watch my mother go through more pain.

We presumed it was a secondary cancer, which is somewhat scarier than primary cancer. Primary cancers can be removed quite easily these days, and the prognosis is pretty good. If you are still clear after five years of monitoring, then it usually means that you are completely free of cancer. If a secondary appears during this five-year window, it means the cancer has spread, and this requires a more aggressive treatment. When my mother had her first cancer removed, she fortunately did not require any radiation or chemotherapy. She was monitored for five years, and all was clear.

There is still little understood about how the BRCA2 gene behaves. It is rare to get a second cancer in a removed breast—close to a 1 percent chance—but they don't know how rare it is yet for gene carriers. So there she was, facing the demon once more, with a little less audacity than the first time. It turned out it was a second primary cancer, which was good news because the cancer had not spread to other organs in her body.

Even though Mum had watched her mother die of breast cancer, she was still surprised that she'd gotten it herself. It was a common belief at the time that breastfeeding reduced your risk of breast cancer. Mum had breast-fed five children, the last one for a staggering three years! So the first time she was diagnosed with breast cancer she was surprised; the second time she was dumbfounded.

When my mother had her first breast cancer surgery, she didn't know she had BRCA2. She only had one breast removed and opted not to have a reconstruction. Ten years later, knowing what she knows now, she wishes she'd had both removed. Ten years after her mastectomy, when she found out she had the BRCA2 mutation, she had her ovaries removed, as this is a recommended procedure for carriers of the gene mutation. Mum had already been through "the change," so it was pretty straightforward. She really wanted to remove her other breast but was put into a predicament. It turned out the heart surgery she'd been awaiting for so long was imminent, and this took priority over the removal of her healthy breast. But first they had to remove the new cancer.

The four months of surgeries my mother endured before Christmas 2007 read like a horror story. She had her ovaries removed, then her second breast cancer removed, then open-heart surgery to replace a mitral valve, and finally twelve weeks of radiation. There was only one moment, a fleeting glimpse, where I felt my mother's eyes silently pleading that enough was enough, that she was tired of trying to survive. I had never seen her so frail. But as I said, it was fleeting, and if you ask her about that moment, she would heartily deny it. When I say my mother is as strong as an ox, I really mean she's as strong as ten thousand oxen on steroids! In the end, my mother's chest looks like a disastrous road map that leads to a little place called "I'm still here," and we are so glad.

Scientific knowledge of how these gene mutations behave and what affects them is still in its infancy. There is still the risk that my mother's breast cancers could recur, which seems to be a possible characteristic of the BRCA2 mutation, but we can only take one step at a time as we all navigate this uncharted territory.

8

meeting dr. d

For better or for worse, ethically right or wrong, I now had the BRCA2 knowledge implanted in my brain. I was armed with information that could affect my mortality within ten years. I could not have it removed, forget about it, or even just ignore it; I had to deal with it.

I let things settle for a few months after the genetics counselor outlined some of my options, and then I set about doing my own research.

First, I found varying statistics about my risks. I guessed that because the BRCA2 had only been discovered in 1995, there was a scarcity of data on the risks and management of women who are gene positive. Conservative risks were as low as 40 to 60 percent, but then I was informed it was between a 65 and 80 percent risk over a lifetime. The risk for ovarian cancer ranged from 20 to 60 percent. There is also confusion about lifetime risk because gene carriers predominantly get their breast cancers much younger than the general population of women. I soon abandoned trying to gauge my exact risk and looked to the patterns in my own lineage, still trying to keep the perspective that genes are not the whole story and they are not necessarily our destiny. My family history was pretty damning. The cancer seemed to appear around forty-nine years of age in each generation, sparing only the men.

I kept asking myself, "Do I feel lucky?" Was I going to be one of the few who had the BRCA2 gene mutation and did not go on to develop breast cancer? Ordinarily I would say yes. I have been known to be annoyingly optimistic, and this has served me well. I have survived and, in fact, made a reliable living as an actor for twenty years in an industry that purports 90 percent unemployment. That requires a certain tenacity and optimism that scoffs at daunting statistics. However, there were three things that were testing that optimism in this particular case.

One was that I had seen my mother be not only optimistic but also adamant that she would never get breast cancer. She was sure all the breastfeeding she did for ten years straight would protect her. Now, this may be the case for those who are not gene carriers, but the BRCA2 factor was not taken into account, and it seems the breastfeeding did not protect her. She was also positive that once she had her breast completely removed, the cancer would not come back, especially a whole decade later. But again, the gene mutation was not factored into this equation.

There was a prevailing idea in my mother's and previous generations that women who worry too much and repress their anger bring on their own breast cancer: the cancer personality. This unproven theory angered me so much, but I know it drove my mother to actively "unworry." To my knowledge, my grandmother was a noble and strong woman, and if my mother was any tougher, she would rust. I rail at the thought that they in any way suffered breast cancer because of some psychological weakness. For me, the BRCA2 gene is tangible proof that breast cancer is a scientifically based disease of the body, not of a person's character. I like this pragmatism that BRCA2 brings.

Another thing that tested my "do I feel lucky?" attitude was the presence of my son. He was still so little—only four years old—and my instinct and desire as a mother was to nurture and protect him for as long as I possibly could. This drove me to seek choices that were practical and concrete. Kaspar actually made up a song for me on his guitar one day, unprompted by any talk of breast cancer, as I had not discussed it with him as yet. The song went, "Mummy, please don't die before me, please stay alive for all my life." Great!

I did not have the choice to do nothing because I could not "unknow" what I now knew. My cousin, who chose not to have the test in spite of the fact that she has a fifty–fifty chance of being a gene carrier, had the opportunity to do nothing. I respected this choice and think it is, in one way, providing her with an easier opportunity to be positive because she is dealing with better odds. I no longer had the luxury to be blissfully ignorant. If I could go back and make the choice again whether to have the test or not, I would still do it, but I understand those who don't. I feel there is a very fine line between positive thinking and denial. So about five months after my BRCA2 confirmation, I decided to make an appointment with a breast cancer specialist.

Enter Dr. Daniel de Viana, a handsome, young doctor.

I loved him instantly. He was so honest and clear and balanced about my situation, and he had such shiny skin and sparkly eyes, which are very good qualities for a breast cancer doctor.

He explained that I had three choices. The first was to engage in rigorous monitoring, including six-monthly mammograms, six-monthly ultrasounds, a yearly MRI, and a yearly ovarian ultrasound and CA-125 blood test. These tests are used as surveillance to detect any changes as early as possible. They are not infallible; cancer could begin to grow any time in the months between your last test and the next.

Annual mammography is now standard practice for women in the general public who are over fifty years of age. However, for carriers of a gene mutation, there is no precise age when monitoring should start. He told me the cancer could appear at any age, even though in my history it usually appeared at around age forty-nine. The difficulty with younger women having mammograms is that breast tissue is denser, and it makes it a little harder to detect small cancers, hence the addition of ultrasound, which can detect small tumors that are missed by mammograms. The breast MRI is much more sensitive than both ultrasound and mammography in young women, detecting 64 to 100 percent of breast cancers. Sometimes, though, this machine is a little too sensitive and can give false positive results, causing unnecessary biopsies.

What Dr. D outlined seemed like a thorough regimen that would make me feel well-covered should any cancer begin to grow. Then, of course, swift treatment could begin.

One of my considerations in taking the surveillance option would be finances. After my consult with Dr.

D, he sent me off to have a mammogram, ultrasound, blood test, and ovarian ultrasound. I spent an entire day on the phone trying to find a place that would bulk bill my mammogram. I was shocked to find that they didn't exist anymore. Unless you were over fifty, you had to pay between 180 and 300 dollars, with up to 100 dollars being refunded by Medicare. I argued on the phone that I had a predisposition to breast cancer because of a BRCA2 gene mutation, but no one knew what I was talking about. Finally I found a place that would bulk bill. The lady on the phone had no idea about any gene mutations—I think she thought I was a little delusional and felt sorry for me.

Unfortunately Dr. D was not happy about me having my mammogram there because only one radiographer views the scan, and Dr. D insists on two, as do most specialists. Well, this was just the beginning. The ultrasound cost me 175 dollars with an 85-dollar refund, and the ovarian ultrasound cost 180 dollars with a refund of 85 dollars. Forget the MRI—I would never be able to afford one at 345 to 700 dollars with no refund at all. Then add all this to Dr. D's specialist fee twice a year to check the results. When I thought about paying these large sums of money twice a year for the rest of my life, I felt pretty powerless. I knew I literally would not be able to afford it.

As these gene tests were still quite new, my case fell into an unknown crack. From what I have seen, if you're diagnosed with breast cancer, the Medicare system supports you very well. I, of course, did not have breast cancer, but it was essential for my survival that I have these tests, which are yet to be recognized as being essential. I'm sure things will change as the governments and medical systems catch up with science, but I was caught between the proverbial rock and a hard place.

I did have private health insurance, but only the very basic coverage. Being an actor may seem glamorous, but most of us hover precariously close to the poverty line. If you don't believe me, next time you happen to be invited to the opening night of a show, watch the actors as they come out for the post-show party—they run straight for the food table. It's true; I do it all the time. We are underpaid and have such limited work opportunities in this country. But what price can you put on your health? If I took the surveillance option, I would just have to find a way to earn more money.

Another important consideration when choosing the surveillance option is that it is not preventive. There is a high likelihood that BRCA2 carriers will get cancer, and once you have it, there is a strong likelihood you will get subsequent cancers, be they secondary or multiple primaries. If you are unfortunate enough for cancer to become a reality, you will have to undergo surgeries to save your life and then possibly radiation and chemotherapy. If I accepted this surveillance option, I would have to be fully prepared for the possible side effects of these treatments—early menopause, hair loss, and pain and discomfort.

Another element of the surveillance option was living life almost "waiting for cancer." How would you *not* think about it constantly? Would my daydreams of running through the Tuscan countryside with the obligatory Italian lover have to accommodate the possibility of a head scarf and no breasts? Should I be practical in my fantasies as a way to accept the inevitable?

The second choice I had was to take a drug called Tamoxifen that was being tested to find out if it could prevent breast cancer in women at high risk. At this stage, the drug has been proven to reduce the risk of cancer by 50 percent in women in the general population, but it is not yet proven to work in BRCA carriers. The disadvantages of this drug are that it may cause menopausal symptoms and increase the risk of uterine cancer, cataracts, and blood clots.

My third choice was to have a prophylactic mastectomy, which is the preventive removal of both breasts. Current research shows it reduces the risk of developing breast cancer by over 90 percent, so my chance of developing the disease would fall below the 10 percent risk, which is the same as the general population of women with no genetic mutation. It is major surgery and carries all the related risks. If you choose to reconstruct, there is loss of sensation in the reconstructed breasts and an inability to breastfeed, plus the complicated cosmetic issues.

Again one of the factors is the cost. With my private health coverage and after all refunds, factoring in reconstruction, I would be spending out of pocket around 10,000 dollars and would be losing about twelve weeks' income for the recovery time from two surgeries. This would seem comparable to the cost of surveillance, but in fact, it turns out to be the cheaper option over a lifetime. But with this choice of the prophylactic mastectomy comes the strange, overwhelming psychological predicament of removing two perfectly healthy breasts.

I discussed with Dr. D the possibility of exploring alternative therapies. Of course, as a medical practitioner, he wouldn't offer me advice on this; however, he did say there is no right or wrong choice. He reiterated the importance of surveillance while I decided.

My head was swimming with statistics, risk factors, and probabilities. As I said good-bye to Dr. D, assuring him I would have my scans done, do breast self-examination, and see him in six months' time, he smiled his blameless smile.

9

chrissy's decision

Meanwhile, my sister Christine, after receiving her positive test, was struggling with her own decision. She felt confused, and silly for feeling confused. As we shared our feelings of mutual confusion at this time, we often thought of Elsie and Maude and how ridiculous it was that we were window-shopping for ways to treat our not-yet-present breast cancer. What would they be thinking? What would they do?

It's strange that until a few years ago we had never heard of the BRCA2 gene and now it seemed to be everywhere, like something suddenly coming into fashion: the new black. "Oh yeah, I've got one of those." It is such a unique and exciting time in history because we have deciphered the entire human genome and predictive testing is becoming more widely available. However, exciting is not a term I would use for finding out you will probably get cancer, just not yet. I found myself in an unprecedented predicament, surrounded by all the women in my family who shared the same questions, fears, and bewilderment, wondering what we would do with this information.

In a macabre coincidence, just when Christine received her positive BRCA2 result she also received a call from her close friend Sue Bradley in Perth. Without mincing words, Sue told her she had breast cancer and was about to undergo a radical mastectomy. Christine flew to Perth to be with her friend.

Sue has been one of Chrissy's closest friends for the last twenty years. Her family, like ours, has a high incidence of breast cancer, carried through from her father's side. Sue's older sister was diagnosed with breast cancer in her twenties and had a double mastectomy. Hence Sue was quite aware that it was important to keep an eye out. Sue, who is now fifty, had been having mammograms yearly for the last decade. When she was forty-eight, she actually missed her mammogram but remembered to have one the following year. It was in this forty-ninth year that a lump was detected and confirmed to be cancer.

When Sue was in the hospital for her mastectomy, Chrissy encouraged her to ask for the gene test. Sue also asked that they remove both of her breasts, not just the one that had a tumor. The surgeon was reluctant to do this because the other breast seemed clear of cancer, but Sue was adamant. When they did the double mastectomy, they found that the other breast was also riddled with cancer.

Sue's gene test came back positive for BRCA2. This prompted her sister to immediately have the test, which also proved positive. Both sisters, both with BRCA2, and both having been diagnosed with breast cancer, decided immediately to have full hysterectomies.

The gene test gave Sue the fighting spirit to try to

prevent cancer from affecting her ovaries. The BRCA2 gene had already claimed her breasts and her sisters', and she wasn't willing to allow it to invade any more body parts.

Sue had a difficult time with the double mastectomy and chemotherapy. She had decided that she wanted reconstruction. Sue, like me, was single, and I think that has a big influence on the decision of whether or not to have reconstruction. Her sister, on the other hand, had chosen not to reconstruct all those years ago and has been content to simply wear prosthetics.

Nursing Sue through part of her recovery was empowering for Chrissy and helped her to decide on a strategy for her own future. When she returned from Perth, Chrissy was determined to go ahead with a prophylactic mastectomy. She is eighteen months older than I am and felt she was short of time to take any other course of action. She had, of course, seen Dr. D, done her research, and watched some pretty horrific videos of the procedure. She did not want to get breast cancer. She did not want to go through what Sue was going through. She saw Sue at her worst, and for Chrissy it was a no-brainer; if she had an opportunity to avoid Sue's fate, she would.

I'm not saying this decision was an easy one for her. She was scared—very scared—but ultimately knew it was the right thing for her to do. Her son David, who is twenty-four, made himself clear that he thought she should have the mastectomy. He did not want his mom to get breast cancer. The medicos, clinicians, and counselors were careful not to influence our decision in any way, but at some point I know I was screaming out for someone to tell me what to do. I was so confused. People around us all had opinions about what we should do and what they would do in the situation, and I appreciated the advice, but ultimately it had to be my own decision.

Those closest to us passionately put their argument forward because they loved us so much. It was crazy, though, when people who hardly knew us heard a brief summary of the situation and offered their two bits' worth based on myopic beliefs. Comments ranged from, "Oh, you're not going to cut your breasts off, are you? Gross!" to "I wouldn't wait; you could have cancer right now. You'd be an idiot to wait. What are you waiting for, you idiot?" It was quite an interesting time, and regardless of the plethora of unwanted feedback, I couldn't help it: I found myself offering up the topic for discussion on many occasions, sometimes provocatively and inappropriately.

One night Chrissy, Elisha, and I went out on the town simply to ask total strangers what they thought. I'm not really sure why we did this, but it is quite a Neave thing to do, when faced with difficulty, to try to wring as many laughs out of the situation as possible before we have to get serious and grown-up about it.

Once Chrissy had made her decision, she was quick to put it all into action. She booked her surgery for August 2007, arranged time off work, and prepared herself for this life-changing event. It was almost as if she wanted it to happen really quickly so she wouldn't get scared and change her mind. She had the full support of her family, but I knew that ultimately the drama between her femininity and sense of mortality would be one she needed to play out on her own.

10

procrastination

While Chrissy exercised certainty, I procrastinated whenever possible. I spent a good deal of time flitting around, trying to cover as much ground as I could, researching all aspects of cancer and genetics. I'm not sure if I was exploring options or developing strategies to defend myself at every turn against comments and opinions from others. The BRCA2 gene seemed so concrete to me. It was real, it was inside me, and even though we have yet to understand how and why it does what it does, it was a little time bomb ticking away. So why was I making appointments with alternative therapists who would press against my arm and try to make me confess to some deep and gripping anxiety about something that happened to me as a fetus? Not sure, but I did it, and it was an adventure.

I sat in front of an Indian swami who believed that disease is a state of "dis-ease" in the body. Many times in my life I have successfully sought nonmainstream answers to medical situations, but this was a big medical situation, and the stakes were quite high. I wanted clarity and no nonsense. As the swami spoke to me for over an hour, Kaspar got bored and fell asleep on my chest, and somehow the swami drew a correlation, "See, this is where the whole problem emanates from, a mother is so nurturing and giving that it depletes her, right there in her chest area." My eyes narrowed; if loving my son less was going to save my life, I was a goner.

On a different bent, I attended the 11th International Congress on Human Genetics and listened to eminent scientists. I asked questions of these science geeks with such erudition that I could have been mistaken for a geek myself. It was all very impersonal, though, and I felt a definite canyon between the research of genetics and the human face of it all—how all these progressions in science were being translated into the lives of real people, like me, for example.

I also researched epigenetics as much as one of my intellectual standing could. I definitely had enough clarity to understand that genes are not the entire story. So if this is the case, where is the rest of the manuscript? Epigenetics at this point is suggesting that genes not only must be present but also need to be switched on or off, and nobody quite knows how this happens yet. Scientists believe that activating or deactivating genes has a lot to do with the environment that the cell is in. The environment could mean your diet and lifestyle but also the combination of other genes in your body that may be enablers or disablers.

I think this branch of science will eventually complete the picture regarding our genes and how they work. It's fascinating, but it really just refers to the ever-present question of nature versus nurture. Genes do not necessarily dictate everything. They may dictate a person's potential, but science adheres to the fact that this same potential may be changed or enhanced by environmental influences.

The discovery of this information confused me even more, however, because in my case, four generations of women whose cells all lived in completely different environments had a BRCA2 gene that switched on at the same age in their very different lives. Or is it that internal environments are also passed down to our children—in the way we think, how we bring up our children, and what they in turn do for their children? I always remember a peculiar moment I had with my mother when I was about seventeen. I had moved out of home and was at university, and my mother was helping me to move into a new flat. I was folding towels, and Mum said, "That's not how you fold towels." And I said, "Yes, this is how I fold towels, Mum." She replied anxiously, "No, no, that is not how you are supposed to fold towels." My dander was up. "Mum, I am a grown-up now, and I can fold my towels whatever way I wish. Now, I know how you fold towels, and I actively decided to do it differently because I am my own person with my own way of folding towels." Mum was a little distressed now. "But you don't understand. The way you're folding that towel is the way that my mother folded her towels, and I tried to change too and fold my own way and now you're doing it her way!" I've always wondered about this inherited towel trait that tried to skip a generation.

There are currently more questions than answers on whether genes are, in fact, our destiny. Can we switch off our genes through the power of thought? Can God switch off my genes if I pray enough? Looking for answers, and without a lot of time, I made an appointment with a naturopath who suggested that there could be something about the aging process in my family history that activated this gene. Quite likely, but how was I going to hold back the aging process in my body? It was already in full swing.

I certainly could take control of certain environments that my cells lived in. I have always been healthy and fit, I've practiced yoga for many years, I don't drink very much or take drugs, and I use as many chemical-free products in my house and on my body as my purse strings will allow (except for the crystal deodorant, which had no effect on my smelly armpits). I'm the one in the family who everyone calls the tree-hugging, Tibet-freeing hippy. I just laugh at this because I'm really not nearly as conscious of these things as I would like to be. I would like to be more embracing of a holistic lifestyle, but I am a bit lazy.

I was concerned, though, that if I tried radical diet and lifestyle changes as a preventive measure, this little gene would just laugh at me. Not that I was giving all the power to this gene, but it was tangible, it was real, and it was potentially dangerous. I could find little to match the power of this gene's track record in my family.

I found a fantastic website called FORCE: Facing Our Risk of Cancer Empowered. Devouring their articles, information, and personal stories was, as it suggests, empowering. I realized that I was well informed through the avenues I had researched.

While exploring alternate routes, I heard the story of

a woman who found out she had breast cancer and chose not to have a mastectomy because she wanted to try to cure herself. This is a life choice that I would not normally judge, but as it was, she died slowly and in front of her two small children. My maternal instinct jumped in and damned her for it. She would possibly still be alive and with her kids if she chose surgery. I was shocked at my reaction; I guess I was projecting myself into her position and could not reconcile my ethical choices over and above that of my duty as a mother.

At the same time as I was foraging away, trying to find palpable answers, I was being enriched by endless discussions on the mysteries of life. The nature of our human condition illuminates little bits of itself in times of real crisis, and choices we make at that time will only reveal themselves to be right or wrong once the entire tapestry of our lives is formed. Whether they are the choices we should have made or not we will only be able to judge for ourselves. I learned that I am actually not afraid of death, I guess because I was not actually dying and this was still theoretical.

My mother consciously always talked to us of death so we wouldn't be afraid. She said she did this because she suspected the history of cancer in our family was more than just coincidence. We traveled the country a lot as kids on family driving holidays. Our parents insisted on showing us as much of this beautiful country in the old Valiant Charger as they could, even though we all had terrible trouble with car sickness and vomited relentlessly on each other. The first thing I remember we would do whenever we pulled up into a new town was visit the cemetery. My mother loved cemeteries, and we all grew to love them too. We would run around and find the oldest grave, the funniest name, and the prettiest headstone. I still find great peace in cemeteries and often take the Sunday papers and a takeaway latté to my local cemetery just to relax.

But dying is so inevitable I'm perplexed that we are ever surprised by it. I'm puzzled by the surprise people express when they hear someone has cancer. Maybe because I have been around it so long, I see it as just the human rust, a part of life. Also our obsession with trying to stay alive, to cheat death, worries me. But is this not exactly what I was trying to do?

11

a documentary
. . . .
and a decision

Things seemed to go back to normal for all of us for a while after the helter-skelter of the six months since our genetic findings. It was as if we had been invaded by the knowledge of BRCA2 and now were just an occupied territory surrendering for the time being, knowing the struggle for emancipation was to come. It was July 2007, and Chrissy went back to the office, waiting to have her surgery in August. I had several shows to do and a decision to make, and Elisha had several years before she needed to make a decision. Mum had had her second cancer removed, her ovaries out, and then open-heart surgery, and she was about to begin twelve weeks of radiation.

I was in a privileged position in that I was going to see my sister go through the very surgery I was contemplating. Chrissy was terrified. There was no precedent for her other than a frightening video she viewed at Dr. D's about breast cancer and reconstruction. She saw her friend Sue during her ordeal, but Sue was a cancer patient and Chrissy was not. Perhaps if you're a cancer patient, having your breasts removed might bring some relief, but my sister had two healthy breasts, and they were soon to be gone.

When I first went to see the genetic counselor, she planted a small seed in my head that niggled away at me. She mentioned that because I was an actor, I should make a documentary on my BRCA2 story. I gave it no more thought at the time because the small tsunami that the gene was causing in my family made it hard to see the wood for the trees. However, as my research slowly revealed, there was very little information to help support people like me and my sisters emotionally while we made the enormous decisions we were being forced to make. There were plenty of statistics and scientific equations, but there was a shortage of resources that helped give a human face to the rapidly evolving science that was affecting real lives.

I made numerous calls to breast cancer clinicians, institutions, and research centers to ascertain if, in their opinion, such a documentary would be useful in helping people navigate the narrow corridors of gene identification. There was a resounding "yes," and I almost felt a duty to use my situation to help the community at large. Because within just one family—our family—there was such a high concentration of positive BRCA2 women, it seemed as though we could be representative of the general public.

It was a good idea, but how to make it a reality was

beyond me. Then out of left field, my brother Denny stepped up and said, "Well, are we going to make this documentary or not?" Denny was a moderately successful businessman by now, and he was wise and careful with his money. Whenever one of the family got in a bother financially, we could always count on Denny to rescue us if needed; he was far from a scrooge, but he was not reckless. Why on earth would he want to put his hard-earned money into making a documentary about his mom and three sisters and their bothersome boobs? But he put the ball in motion, invested most of his savings, hired a crew, bought a huge camera, and produced his first-ever documentary.

It had not occurred to me that perhaps Denny; my other brother, John; and my father were a little freaked out that all of their womenfolk were dealing with this potentially life-threatening situation. The BRCA2 gene can, of course, be passed to the boys, but with only small elevations in risks for cancer. I realized the offer from my brother to make the documentary was an emotional response that made him feel as though he was doing something rather than just standing by watching.

So for the next four weeks, we had a camera in our faces trying to capture the complexity of the choices we were making. The camera would follow Chrissy's operation to remove her healthy breasts. She was so open and natural in front of the camera, and I was proud of her for sharing this frightening experience in order to make it less frightening, hopefully, for others.

In true Neave style, we decided to have a breast plaster casting night—a united front—in support of our valiant champion, Chrissy, who would go forth on our behalf. We had bought kits for pregnant women to make plaster casts of their bellies, and we simply applied the plaster a little higher. I think we all wanted to freeze a moment in time where our bodies were all still our own—for posterity, perhaps—something more tangible than a photograph or a faded memory. There was wine and pasta and a sea of plaster all over my otherwise extremely tidy house. There was also a camera, a director, and a sound operator that were now part of the furniture, which we found very easy to ignore.

The night was hilarious. Mum wanted us to make subtle enhancements on her one remaining breast, which took all of my limited sculpting prowess. Elisha, who openly declares she has "PNP" (perfect nipple placement, for those like me who are not in the know), was distraught when one of her plaster nipples collapsed. I tried to remold it using a caper. Chrissy's went off without a hitch, but by the time they got to doing mine, it was about midnight, everyone except me was hammered, and the novelty had worn off somewhat.

Things got shoddy. I had plaster all over my face, and my plaster boobs were suffering from too much wine and complacency. I was mad, to my surprise, because I wanted them to look just right so if I decided to remove my breasts, I would have proof that they had been extremely nice breasts. When everyone left, I found myself beavering away trying to perfect my cast with a little bowl of water and scraps of bandage. After a while this seemed a little desperate and unsettling, so I let go of perfection and went to bed.

Each of us painted our busts according to our own tastes. Mum had her two youngest grandchildren paint hers, and it looked so colorful and random in a beautiful and innocent way. Chrissy's had a forties' touch with a heart in the middle made out of old lace. Elisha's was perfectly her: bright pink and covered in diamantes. Mine I painted gold and then aged with a fake oxidized look, leaving it looking just like a classical Greek sculpture. They were all fabulous, and we were so glad we did it.

On the Saturday night before Chrissy's Monday surgery, we had a "farewell to her breasts" party. I made a sponge cake carved into two breasts with pink icing and strawberries for nipples. The sponge burned black, but I disguised it with extra icing. The cold strawberries slid slowly off the breasts as the night went on, leaving two gutters in the icing trailed with red. I threw the untouched cake into the bin after everyone had left.

My brother Denny gave a little speech about how proud he was of his sisters and that together we were going to raise awareness for BRCA gene carriers. He began to cry and could not go on with his speech. All of us girls rushed to hug him, but I was shocked by his emotional response. He is always so strong and together. I have never seen my brother lose his temper or his nerve like the rest of us are always doing. Of all of the family, he is the most levelheaded; he is the rock, the one who can sweep in and fix everything with great efficiency. But he was scared for his sisters and perhaps felt guilty that we had to bear the burden of this gene mutation while he could only stand by and watch. Well, he wasn't just watching. He was going to be helping the entire BRCA population with his documentary.

Chrissy was not in a partying mood, which is unusual for her but not surprising considering the circumstances.

I think she just wanted to be quietly alone with her husband and her boobs. I guess the time for laughing it off and squeezing comedy out of the situation was ending and we now had to face a more sober reality.

The camera filmed Chrissy the night before her surgery and was with her on the actual day. I think in a strange way this helped Chrissy to feel less alone. The documentary and its possible service to others made her feel she was doing something important and bigger than just herself. I think it added a little excitement for her too and perhaps was a distraction from the anxiety.

Chrissy's surgery took about five hours, during which Dr. D removed as much breast tissue as possible through incisions in her nipples; Chrissy had chosen to keep her skin and nipples. I have to say, it was not pretty in the least to see her flat and bruised torso with several drainage tubes coming out where her proud breasts used to be. When she came to, she said she felt like a house was on her chest, making it hard for her to breathe. She caught sight of her son, David, who was holding her hand, and in a drugged and slurred attempt she asked, "I've made you happy?" To which he replied, "Yes." "Good," said Chrissy, "now go and get a job!"

She went home after five days and spent about six weeks recovering.

After a few days at home, I drove Chrissy to a conference about gene carriers and their options. She was in so much pain I thought I had made a mistake taking her out, but I hoped it would be good for her to talk to other women who perhaps were going through what she was experiencing. I also thought it would help me decide my fate. The conference taught us little that we didn't already know because it seems our own research had been very thorough. What was good, or so I thought, was that Chrissy spoke with a woman who'd had the same surgery but was now at the reconstruction phase. They quickly raced off to the toilet for a show and tell.

I met women who introduced themselves as "Mary, BRCA2" and "Sophie, BRCA1." There was a lot of talk at the conference, not only about breasts but also about ovaries because both BRCA1 and BRCA2 carry a high ovarian cancer risk. Most women there had had their ovaries removed. Chrissy and I were the youngest there and had yet to even think about our ovaries.

I met a woman who was BRCA1 and had had her ovaries removed, but who didn't have medical insurance and couldn't afford to have her breasts removed even though she thought it was more than necessary. This disturbed me and made me realize that because prophylactic surgeries are considered elective, some people have no choice but to wait around and get the cancer before free treatment can be sought. There was a great doctor at the conference, Dr. Paul Belt, who had decided to treat all BRCA1 and 2 carriers without charging the health fund gap, which made it a little less scary financially. Still, without insurance, the hospital stay and all the other charges are debilitating.

Chrissy was fading, and so I took the cue to leave. On the way home, she told me she hated seeing that lady's breasts. She said, "They looked awful. Just two hard lumps stuck to her chest." Chrissy showed her chest in return and felt she was frowned upon for keeping her nipples, which the other lady had not done. She said, "I was made to feel vain because I kept my own nipples!" She was tired and emotional and not in the mood to split hairs over nipples in public toilets with strangers.

I had to relocate to Sydney for a few months to rehearse a new show. I felt bad leaving Chrissy at this time, but I knew she had a lot of support around her. When I spoke to her on the phone, she talked of a lot of pain but mostly grief. After being home for about one week, she began to cry and could not stop. She cried all day and all night. To some extent, emotions can be exacerbated by the after-effects of anesthetics, but the crying went on so long it could no longer be attributed to the drugs. She told me she was okay with her chest being flat and it was not the look of it that bothered her; she just had inexplicable grief she could not control.

Another unexpected reaction for her was a sense of guilt. She felt guilty because she had not had cancer and therefore had no right to feel upset. Many people around her called her brave, but she felt cowardly compared to the women who had to fight for their lives. The crying lasted for about two weeks, and although she had the undying support of her husband, Ray, and her son, David, it was a lonely and inconsolable time.

Chrissy also mentioned that there had been so much excitement and commotion with the cameras around and the filming for the documentary, but as soon as her surgery was over, all that disappeared, and she was not distracted anymore. We'd made a huge fuss over her and then in a split second scattered back into the corners of our own lives and left her alone and flat-chested.

I still had to make a decision. I was procrastinating. But finally I realized I was trying to make a choice that would be satisfactory to others. I wanted to make a choice that would be alternative and brave and defy science and history, that would make the hippies happy and the medicos marvel. I wanted to be the person who said, "No! I believe that I will not get cancer." But I wasn't that person.

I was a mother, and I was practical. I believed that there was only a very slight chance that I wouldn't get cancer. I believed that if I waited for the cancer to arrive, I would end up having a mastectomy and then worry for the rest of my life that the cancer could have spread and that I would potentially have to fight the harder fight of secondary cancer. I decided that although I would definitely die one day, I would try to extend my life a little and have the preemptive mastectomy.

I'm not sure how long it took for me to make my decision, but after seeing Chrissy's surgery, I knew I had to do the same. It was an enormous relief when I finally had a definite strategy. I booked my surgery for July 2008, about eight months away. I had to find a gap in my work schedule, and as I am an itinerant, this is both easy and difficult. I am always at the mercy of other people's schedules. Job offers came in that coincided with my surgery, and I had to be strong and say, "No. I'm going to have my breasts removed at that time; I am not available." As an actor in Australia, it is hard to turn down any offers because there are so few jobs around; you just don't say no to anything. A few times I was tempted to take a job and just shift my surgery, but I knew I had to "lock it in" or I would always be shifting it.

Deciding to have a mastectomy was likely to have repercussions in the long term for my work as a physical theater performer. I guess I'm now what is known as a specialist performer—a trained actor who can be called upon to do strange things with her body. I teach a lot of physical theater, trying to get actors to use their whole bodies to tell stories not just their voices and intellect. I still perform for companies that blend dance and theater, so my work can be highly physically demanding, but I mix it up with film work and mainstream theater that is less stressful on my body. No one could really tell me if I could continue to be such an athletic performer after my surgery, but I decided to work on the premise that anything is possible and take it from there.

I was in Sydney working on a show for the 2008 Sydney Festival with Force Majeure. Since I had worked for Force for about eight years, the whole company was aware of my situation and subsequently my decision to go ahead with the surgery. When creating works for Force, we always draw on our own personal experiences where possible, so my director, Kate, was keen for me to incorporate the whole breast cancer thing if we could. So there was no getting away from it. I was attempting to wring advantage from adversity. This little BRCA2 gene had not only weaseled its way into our lives, but now it was also getting a spot on the Sydney Opera House stage—what a megalomaniac.

A strange thing was happening to my breasts at this time: they were getting bigger. I have always had fairly small breasts, except for the breastfeeding year, when things blew all out of proportion. But my breasts are generally smallish and easily overlooked. Suddenly people were looking, commenting, and generally admiring them. The people I had known for a long time were more up-front about it, making comments like, "Wow, what's going on with your breasts? They're huge!"

In the last year, I had talked about my breasts endlessly, and when you talk about a part of your body, your hand unconsciously touches that body part. I wondered if they were just becoming overstimulated. There was lots of poking and prodding from doctors, and I think maybe my breasts were liking it—not me consciously, but my breasts—and they were out of my control. Although I was single—almost pathologically single by now—I was not so desperate that I looked forward to my mammograms. Seriously, how archaic to put your breast in a metal vice—it truly is an apparatus of torture, not pleasure. So with ever-expanding breasts, without any medical or rational reason, I put it down to a "force majeure" and went out and bought new bras.

12

to reconstruct *or*

· ·

not to reconstruct?

With my breasts now putting on the performance of their lives, it was hard to be objective about my next decision, which was whether to have a reconstruction or not. If you really think about it, a woman's breasts have no biological function unless you are planning to have more children. I am fairly certain that, at thirty-nine and single, I won't be having any more kids. I am blessed to have the one I have, and he is perfect.

I had experienced the bliss of breastfeeding. That's when my breasts first made real sense; they were filled with nourishing milk that made my baby thrive. I loved breastfeeding so much. I had one of those feeding chairs that rocked gently and a matching ottoman. At night in Kaspar's room, with the fairy lights on the window, I would feed and rock and listen to "Pachelbel's Canon" and stare lovingly at this little angel at my breast. I didn't want it to end. I cried when he was weaned.

So now they just sat there, not really doing much. If you have a leg or hand amputated, it is obvious you need some sort of reconstruction or prosthesis to continue to function as normally as possible. But my breasts didn't do anything practical; they just made me look normal and feel feminine. In terms of evolution, when we began to walk upright, our breasts developed in such a way as to attract a mate. Previously, when on all fours, it was our bums in the air that did all the attracting. Thank goodness for evolution. So my breasts still had the purpose of attracting a mate, I suppose. But did I need plastic boobs to find love at this stage of my life? Now that I'm older, I have experience, a developed intellect, skills, and a myriad of other gifts that only come wrapped with age. I would hate to think that it all comes down to what is or isn't in my bra.

Our bodies are temporal, and if the time for my breasts and me to be together had expired, I had to think about where my true femininity really resided. If I had reconstruction, the breasts would be artificial, so although I'd look normal from the outside, it would only be a simulated femininity. So I wanted to be sure about who I was getting the reconstruction for. Reconstruction would entail subsequent surgery and recovery time and, of course, would cost money. Reconstruction after mastectomy is nothing akin to breast enhancement—do not be fooled. It is not a boob job. If a woman decides to have breast augmentation, she still retains breast tissue, so the breasts are hers and she has normal sensations, they're just a bit bigger or smaller. Reconstruction is a different story.

There are a few options for reconstruction, depending

on what particular mastectomy you are having. My surgeon explained I could have a "subcutaneous, nipple-preserving, prophylactic mastectomy." This entails removing as much breast tissue as possible while leaving in place all the skin and the nipple. This would allow for a reconstruction that looked a little more natural but would ever so slightly increase your reduced risk of breast cancer because more breast tissue is likely to get left behind than if you take the nipple and skin away. The increased risk is only about 1 or 2 percent. The reconstruction, then, would entail lifting the pectoral muscles off the chest wall, placing an expander bag under it, having the bag inflated over a few months, and then replacing the expander bag with an implant in what is known as "swap-over surgery."

Having your own nipples and skin has quite a good cosmetic result, but there will be little if any sensation in the breast. When the breast tissue is removed, all the nerves are cut, so there is a prevailing numbness. There is also the risk of tissue necrosis because removing as much breast tissue as possible reduces blood supply to the skin and nipple, and sometimes this causes the tissue to die. Then there are the usual risks associated with implants such as rupture, leakage, capsular contracture, and infection around the implant. However, the pictures I saw were quite good as far as breast impersonation goes.

I found myself feeling ridiculous, thinking again of Maude and Elsie. Would they shake their heads in disbelief, laugh out loud, or flick through the breast renovation catalogue with me, chortling, "Ooh . . . they look nice, don't they?" It would have been surreal for them, but medical advances were at my disposal, and I am eternally thankful.

Another type of reconstruction is flap reconstruction. In this procedure, skin, fat, and muscle from another part of the body are used to create the breast mound. Flap reconstruction surgery is more complex than the expansion method, and recovery time is longer. However, as the breast is created using natural tissue, the results can have a more natural feel and appearance. After this, you can have nipple reconstruction using skin grafts and, later, tattooing to create the desired color.

If I decided not to have reconstruction, I would simply have a total mastectomy. This gives the surgeon the opportunity to remove more breast tissue than the subcutaneous surgery. However, it is still not possible to remove every single breast cell. In an American study published in 1999, there where 639 women who had preventive mastectomies of both breasts between the years of 1960 and 1993. Of the 639 women, 90 percent chose to have subcutaneous and 10 percent total mastectomy. Seven women went on to develop breast cancer, and these were all women who had subcutaneous surgery. Still, the reduced risk from both surgeries is higher than 90 percent, which means having preventive mastectomy of either kind reduces a woman's chance of developing breast cancer to a percentage less than that of a woman in the general population.

If I chose to have a total mastectomy, what would that mean for me in terms of my body image and sense of femininity? Until I was actually walking around with no breasts at all, I could only speculate. The strange thing is, I could feel my breasts all the time—I mean, without touching them; they were there making me feminine. If they were removed, I would no longer feel them;

the subconscious sensation of my breasts would be gone. This would probably be so even if I had a reconstruction because of prevailing numbness. I may feel a certain weight of the prosthesis but no sensation on the skin or nipple or internally from the nerves. It was a conundrum.

So let's talk about body image. I was fairly sure that I knew myself well enough to assume I could happily and proudly be seen as a woman with no breasts. I have never been that concerned with what people think of me, if you can believe that coming from an actor! It's true I'm concerned when I'm on stage that I'm engaging the audience, but when I'm not working, I couldn't care less what people make of me. Again, though, I had never been in a situation where I was physically outside of the norm. I was just projecting the person I would hope to be if I chose to not reconstruct my breasts. Maybe this was all I could do: hope to be the person I wanted to be and then try to be that person.

Here's a spanner in the works: if I were to go to the beach, would I wear a bikini top? The person I wanted to be wouldn't want to wear strange little triangles over my no-longer-there breasts. Having a total mastectomy means there would be no nipples, just scars across my chest; so being topless would make sense because there is nothing to see. But would it be too confronting for others? To tell the truth, I would normally wear a full sun shirt to the beach anyway; however, if I chose not to reconstruct, I certainly would have to deal with not only my own body issues but also other people's projections.

Okay, there was something else for me to consider: I was almost forty and single. I was almost sure I would want to be with someone who didn't place physical beauty on the top of his list, but it would definitely be an issue—more so than if I was already in a relationship before my surgery.

Chrissy had decided to have reconstruction using the expansion method. The appearance of her breasts is very important to her sense of femininity. Chrissy loves to dress up. She and Ray are obsessed with the 1940s and '50s aesthetic. Their house is like a trip back in time with all their collectibles, but it goes much deeper. As well as running a Lindy Hop dance school with Ray, Chrissy has a Beauty School for Girls business where she does 1940s makeovers for women. This era is very pretty and feminine, with amazing dresses and stockings and gorgeous hairdos, and this is a real reflection of Chrissy. She loves to look good, and she does look good. Reconstruction was a clear choice for her.

Chrissy's friend Sue also chose to reconstruct, using the flap reconstruction technique. The flap reconstruction is supposed to give more of a natural look and feel to the reconstructed breast because it uses a woman's own tissue. Sue did find this to be the case but had trouble coming to terms with the dents left in her back from the donor site. She also had an implant that rotated and had it fixed up with a subsequent surgery.

I went around obtaining opinions from different women on whether they would have reconstruction or not, and the responses were as varied as the women. One friend who has always had huge breasts said she would welcome the relief of a flat chest and probably get a beautiful tattoo that she could fashionably expose. Another friend who has no breasts to speak of said she would definitely use the opportunity to finally have something to put in her bra. My mother thought because of my personality that I could go without breasts, and this obviously would give me the best chance at survival. Mum doesn't even wear a prosthetic in her bra, mainly because she stabbed it with a pitchfork while gardening and couldn't afford to buy another. You can see she only has one breast but, like the lines on her face, it tells the story of who she is and what she has been through.

I was very confused again, but what I was most concerned about was who I would be getting the reconstruction for. Was I trying to make other people feel comfortable or myself? I had a while until my surgery, so I decided to wait and let time work its rich and reliable magic.

I went home for a few days for Christmas and saw Chrissy again. Wow, she looked great! It was about six weeks after her surgery, and all her pain had subsided and her emotions were once again stable. She was off all pain medication and back at work. Over the past six weeks, she had been to Dr. D to have three "pump-ups." Because Chrissy had chosen to have reconstruction, during her surgery Dr. D removed her breast tissue and put in expander bags. These bags go underneath the pectoral muscles to attempt to stretch the muscle in preparation for prosthetics later.

Normally, if a woman has breast implants, they are inserted behind the breast tissue. But when you have no breast tissue, this isn't possible, so they are placed behind the pectoral muscles. To create room for the implants, the whole pectoral muscle is lifted off the chest and some surrounding rib muscles to eventually hold the implant in place. During my acrobatic days, I had, on one occasion, torn my pec muscle, and it was so excruciating I can't imagine how I would cope with the entire muscle inflamed. Chrissy seemed to downplay both the physical and emotional pain, but she had Ray to lean on, and he took much of the weight of her recovery like a perfect partner.

Chrissy's expander bags made her look just like she had breasts when wearing a shirt. Under the shirt, you could see that they were not quite boobs. They had a strange shape—a little bit squarish—but it gave her a sense of normality when out and about.

BRCA2 had edged Chrissy toward a precipice, but thankfully she was now well clear of it. All in all, her surgery was a success and free of complications, and although she still had a swap-over surgery to come in three months, she admitted she felt truly liberated from the worry of breast cancer. It was a great outcome, and I was happy for her and proud of her continued courage.

So Chrissy had bravely paved the way for me to glide on through. I returned to Sydney for more rehearsals and found that because I no longer had to worry about Chrissy and her surgery, I began to anticipate mine. Not a day went by that I didn't contemplate my impending life without breasts. I was filled with contradictory emotions. One part of me looked forward to a little hospital rest, where I could sleep whenever I wanted and finally have time to learn the entire epic poem "The Rime of the Ancient Mariner" by Samuel Taylor Coleridge (all 143 stanzas). The other part of me was filled with terror at the prospect of hating my body from here to eternity.

13

my boobs' last performances

I was now looking at every woman's breasts with a sense of longing and admiration. They truly are amazing: big, small, young, old, pendulous, and pert. I was glad of the opportunity to genuinely appreciate all mammary glands. What is also great is that there is a sisterhood when it comes to breasts. I can say to a girlfriend, "I love the shape of your breasts," and it is totally accepted. She is likely to even let me touch them. But if a man said that, he would probably be considered somewhat of a pervert. I was on a breast awareness campaign, and I was really enjoying it. I observed that when a woman hugs you, she is really just squishing her breasts up against you. Okay, so maybe a hug is about two hearts coming close together, but whatever, the breasts get there first. How astonishing is it when you get a huge hug from a huge-breasted woman. It's like . . . well, it's like being hugged by a huge-breasted woman, and it's great.

I was busy with work right up until my surgery. I had to make a film, direct a children's show, do a physical theater show in Melbourne, and then head straight to the hospital. This was good in so many ways because time went by quickly and I could try to save money. I was going to have to pay for my surgery with my credit card, so I cleared the existing debt. I love my job and I wouldn't be happy doing anything else, but I can work flat out all year and still be on the bread line; so much of the money for the arts goes into infrastructure and administration that only a small portion is left over for the artists.

So I paid about 10,000 dollars for my surgery with my credit card and had no income for the twelve weeks that I'd set aside for recovery. If I'd had a desk job, I'm sure I could have gone back to work sooner, but I couldn't jump back on stage until I had full range of movement and had built up the strength once again in my arms. I was getting ready for some serious debt. Even though I had worked consistently for twenty years after studying for three years and obtaining a degree, I had no such thing as sick leave or long service leave—that's working in the arts. We are contract workers, and when we don't work, we don't get paid. When we do get paid, it's not very much—an average wage for an actor in Australia is 10,500 dollars per annum.

I had the opportunity to make my first feature film, *Girl Clock*, in June 2008. I had really given up the idea of ever having a lead role in a feature film because if it hadn't happened after twenty years, it was probably not likely to. But at the eleventh hour, and before I was too old to play anything but somebody's spinster aunt, someone took a punt on me.

There is so much riding on film and television to make a profit, or at the very least to pay back investors. And these mediums cost so much money it's insane. So usually they have to cast big names or what's called "marquee" actors to give the investors some insurance that the public will recognize someone and want to go to see the film. Trouble is, you can't be a marquee actor until someone, just one person, has given you the chance to be seen in something; they won't cast you if you're unknown, and you're unknown until someone casts you!

When I go to see a film with someone famous in it, it's harder for me to suspend my disbelief that they are actually the character that they are playing. I get distracted by images that I have seen in the tabloids. I remember seeing Emily Watson in *Breaking the Waves*. I had never seen her before, and her portrayal of the character had such a powerful effect on me because she existed only as that character in my mind. She is an extraordinary performer as well, but her anonymity helped me to hear the story in a pure sense.

I'd always had plenty of work as a stage performer, so it never bothered me that the film medium was not very available to me. Then came *Girl Clock*. The director, Jennifer Uzzi, picked me. I'm not sure if the budget allowed for a more famous actor, but who cares? I had been given a chance to do a lead role in a feature film just in the nick of time—while I still had all of my own body parts.

It was a great experience. It was a tight budget, so we worked sixteen-hour days for five weeks. Because I had the main role, I really had to keep the momentum going. If it was 4 a.m. and we were doing a take for the twenty-fifth time and everyone around me was angry and dead on their feet, I still had to pull it out of the bag and give a spot-on performance so that the film would work. I did the best job I could do; I couldn't do any more and I didn't do any less. If I suck, then I was not meant to be a film actor, and I apologize for wasting everyone's money!

When it came time to go to Melbourne for my last show before my surgery, I got some sound advice from my close friend Rachel. I was heading to Melbourne alone; normally Kaspar comes with me when I'm working out of town, but in this instance, he was staying at home with his dad, and I had two weeks flying solo.

The show I was doing was called *Blue Love* at the Malthouse Theatre, and it put me in the perfect light to strut my stuff. My costume was quite saucy, and I wore cool boots that made my legs look fabulous. It was a great show, very physical, and I had to pull off some tricky moves. The only other person in the show was a man, so if there were any single, straight men out there in the audience, the situation was perfect to get their attention.

On opening night, I ventured out into the foyer, hiding behind a glass of free Shiraz for courage, with the full intention of "picking up." I felt ridiculous having this motive in my mind. As the night went on, I found myself terribly alone and just hanging around with a pathetic, desperate feeling inside.

When complaining about my single status at times to close friends, they've remarked that sometimes it can be intimidating to approach me after a show because the performance can put me up on a bit a of a pedestal. Whatever! I just think no one was interested, and I enjoyed feeling sorry for myself all the way home. For the next two weeks, I left the theater out the back door, got takeaway pasta from the restaurant in front of my hotel, and watched documentaries on SBS.

Shaun, my colleague in *Blue Love*, noticed I wasn't quite myself; I was introspective and a little irritable. I apologized to him and explained that I thought it was because my surgery was imminent that I was acting a little strange. I really just wanted to be alone. I did a lot of walking in Melbourne. It was midwinter, and I just walked for miles and miles each day in the bitter cold. It was good because, with the walking and the show, I was going into my surgery feeling very physically fit.

On closing night, I felt strangely elated. It was really happening—the very next week I was having a mastectomy. It's not that I was happy; I think it was fear that was buzzing round my body making me hyper. I was chatting with a friend and her new boyfriend, who asked, "So what are you doing next?" and I blurted out, "Oh, having both of my breasts removed." Poor guy. I had only just met him, but I couldn't help it—it was too good to pass up. I get asked that question all the time as an actor, and I would never get the chance to answer like this again. Of course, the atmosphere plummeted to below zero, and then I had to pay the price for my antisocial confession, which was tedious for them and for me.

14

parting *is such* sweet sorrow

the operation

I had been so busy with work that I hadn't seen much of Chrissy since she had her swap-over surgery. Dr. D removed her expander bags, which had been pumped to her preferred size and left to settle for the last four months. He made incisions under her breasts for this second procedure because her nipples had not liked the last surgery very much. Their blood supply was weak, and Chrissy's circulation had not been that great. Chrissy said it was a breeze compared to the last surgery. She was in the hospital overnight and back at work a week later. The pain was bearable, and she was more than happy with the results. Her breasts looked great. She had opted to increase the size from a B cup to a C cup. You could hardly see any scarring, and if you weren't in the know, they looked like a perfectly normal set of beautiful breasts. The nipples pointed slightly east–west if you wanted to nitpick, but whose breasts are perfect, anyway? She was home and hosed, as they say, and so glad it was all behind her.

By now I had made up my mind to have reconstruction. It just seemed the path of least resistance psychologically. It was going to be far easier for me as an actor, as a woman, and as a relatively young, single woman to have a set of breasts. I don't know why, but I was slightly disappointed in myself for making this decision; I was still partly hanging on to the me that could be the brave cancer "pre-vivor" who refused reconstruction, making a statement that I do not need prosthetics to make me feel normal and feminine. But I also have an uncanny ability to stand by my choices without regret. Now that I was going to have reconstruction, I was going to love my new breasts with all of my might.

I tried to do some preparations at home, knowing I wouldn't be able to do much for a few weeks. I cleaned the house to within an inch of its life. I'm talking serious, cathartic cleaning. When you are pregnant and almost at term, a strange thing happens where you begin to clean the house like a maniac. Most women experience this, and it's a sign that you are about to go into labor. Well, this was even worse. I took down air vents and washed them, pulled apart the wall-mounted air conditioner and cleaned all its moving parts, scrubbed all plug holes with a toothbrush, and sprinkled all mattresses with baking soda and vacuumed them. I don't want to incriminate myself further, but you get the idea; it was madness.

The night before my surgery, Chrissy came over to see

if I was feeling okay. While chatting with her and packing my bag, Kaspar's dad, Sam, came in and said, "I'm feeling really bad that we decided I wouldn't take the day off work tomorrow. I want to come to the hospital and just wait till you're out of surgery." We had previously decided that with Mum and Chrissy, I had enough people coming to the hospital, so Sam should go to work. Besides, his not going would be problematic for his colleagues.

When Sam confessed that he was feeling afraid, I just snapped at him. "Don't be stupid. It's just an operation. I'll be out of it all day. You can't take the day off now, and anyway, it's not all about you!" He defended himself, saying, "Sorry for caring." I blistered something irrational back, which sent him out of the room. Not satisfied, I hurled a few more hurtful comments in his general direction, which then sent him out of the house, leaving me alone with Chrissy and feeling absurd. I looked at Chrissy, and her eyebrows were raised. She said she hadn't ever seen me be so horrible to Sam for no reason at all. I guess I was feeling unnerved.

It's so awful, misdirected anger. As the words are escaping your mouth, you know they're just impostors from the compost of your emotions posing as reasonable arguments. But it's just easier in the end to pretend that they are real rather than backpedal and do what it is you really want to do, which is cry. Shakespeare said it best (Shakespeare always says it best) when Macbeth identifies, "I am in blood steeped so far that to wade no more were as tedious as to go o'er." So I tried to be reasonable and calm as I packed my bag, while those around me dodged my daggers, to continue the *Macbeth* theme.

I had explained to Kaspar that I was going to have an

operation to fix my boobs. It was kind of hard to create images that were not horrifying for a little four-year-old. I think I just said they were going to take out the sick bits and put in some new bits that were not sick. He knows Grandma has only one boob, and he occasionally asks where the other one went. Kids are so reasonable at times of stress and woe. He was not perturbed, and I could tell he felt that he had no cause to worry.

I actually packed the most bizarre things in my hospital bag. In went *The English Parnassus of Epic Poetry* so I could memorize "The Ancient Mariner." I can't honestly say why I have always wanted to learn this poem. There's no question it's full of rich imagery and masterful writing, such as "Water, water everywhere nor any drop to drink," and "Through utter drought all dumb we stood, I bit my arm and sucked the blood and cried, a sail a sail!" But come on. To appreciate it is one thing, to want to learn it means I have some gruesome intent of one day reciting the whole thing to a less-than-enamored audience. Even worse, it will probably be when I'm eighty years old and the grandkids protest: "Mum, please don't make us sit and listen to Granny Ronnie say that long and boring poem about the ship—she spits when she says it and falls asleep in the middle of a sentence and then picks up where she left off!" But in the bag it went, along with an old book on palmistry, which I know nothing about, that's been sitting unread on my bookshelf for years. I also packed a stupid pair of pink scuffs that I never wear because they are too uncomfortable.

When Chrissy had her surgery, she came up with the brilliant idea of getting Mum to make her a few ponchos. Because they go over the head easily, you don't have to lift your arms. It is always cold in hospitals, and she knew that the blanket would be too heavy on her chest. Also you have several drainage tubes coming out of your chest, which makes wearing anything awkward. Mum made her four really cool ponchos in bright pink, leopard print, and cosy, fluffy fabrics. I thought I would just inherit them, but Chrissy donated hers to charity. How quickly we forget. I asked Mum to please make me just one, and it slipped her mind; having a double prophylactic subcutaneous mastectomy was old news in our family. So last into the bag went a pile of totally unwearable clothing.

Inappropriate packing is not a new phenomenon for me. The first time I went to Europe, I put *The Complete Works of William Shakespeare* in my backpack, leaving no room for the Lonely Planet guide. I also took my Rollerblades—not the best for cobbled streets. When I went into labor, my bag consisted of one very unflattering, beige nightie that belonged to my mother. I hate showing photos of Kaspar's first few days in the world. A friend of mine, after giving birth, wore a gorgeous sexy nightie that made her look like the most yummy new mummy in the world. I vow in the future to transform into someone who can pack a bag with class and sensibility.

The next morning, I can honestly say I was looking forward to just getting on with it. I was not afraid, as I trusted Dr. D implicitly, and I had a deep sense that I was doing the right thing. I found it quite exciting checking in, perhaps because I was not sick and also because I have had very few hospital experiences. A hospital is such a hub of activity with so many amazing people looking after you, all of them very skilled and with the uncanny ability to tactfully distract you. It was a beautiful relief to see Dr. D. I think it is very easy to imagine your surgeon as your savior, and for a time, he was the most important man in my life. He was also very charming. Okay, I did mention that I was in a pathologically single state, but I know my sister also developed a healthy crush on Dr. D that lasted until all her surgeries were over. He did the preparations, I wished him luck, and I went to sleep.

The next few days were a haze of drug-induced euphoria. There was certainly a party going on in my head that no one else was invited to. I remember lifting my shirt a lot and showing whoever was around how great my chest looked. I told Sam to take a photo on his phone and send it to a girlfriend of mine in Sydney. A few months later, I saw the photo, and I was nearly sick. There I was, smiling and lifting my shirt, showing off my train wreck of a chest. I had four drainage tubes coming out of what used to be my breasts; it was completely flat, with stitched-on nipples and bruising that went right round to my back. I really couldn't look at the photo—I can't believe I sent it to my poor, unsuspecting friend.

It was at least twenty-four hours before the pain set in. My sister had said she felt like a house was on her chest. I felt cement pylons stacked upon several houses—make that mansions. I mean, I had experienced childbirth—I'm not a complete sook—but this was out of my range. It took morphine, Capadex, and Nurofen at short intervals just to take the edge off the inexorable agony. All the drugs gave me a migraine that caused me to vomit, and this hurt my chest even more.

The most surreal thing happened a few hours after my surgery. Once I was alone, I switched on the television and Oprah was on, which is always somehow comforting when you're in unfamiliar territory. The only time I ever watch Oprah is when I am out of sorts, laid up with the flu, or recovering after a double mastectomy. Well, there she was, reassuring me that the earth was still turning and that there were other people in the world with struggles more horrendous than my own. That day's story was about a forty-year-old woman who'd just had a double prophylactic mastectomy! You can imagine—I thought I was dreaming. I pinched myself, blinked a few times, and watched as her cameras went into an operating room to show the very surgery I'd just had! Thank you, Oprah, for making me feel like I was not alone.

Five days passed in pain and pethidine—the morphine made me too sick. I'm thankful I live in a country where the health system is still reasonably humane. In America, I would have been sent home after one day. I've heard of some women who've been kicked out of the hospital, even against doctors' wishes, because their insurance wouldn't pay for more than one day. They were sent home with bloody tubes coming out of their chests, completely doped after five hours of general anesthetic, and with pain that is terrifying. I could not imagine how detrimental this would be to my recovery and emotional stability. I was so in need of careful attention, and I got it around the clock from those marvelous nurses for five whole days.

Dr. D visited every day and was happy with his work. He also informed me that there were no cancer cells present in the breast tissue they removed, which was reassuring. Chrissy was also found to have no cancer cells present in her breast tissue. Her reaction to this was more complex. She went through a phase of anger at having to have the surgery when there "was no cancer there anyway." If they had found cancer cells, it would have been more tangible proof for her that she had done the right thing.

By the time I was ready to go home, I was as fragile as a thin sliver of glass, again because of the debilitating pain and also because I couldn't use my arms. My pecs were so weak I couldn't take the wrapper off a lolly. I couldn't open doors or dress myself. Someone sent me some flowers, and when the delivery boy handed them to me, I slowly sank to the ground under the weight of this little floral arrangement that seemed to be made of lead. I think the debilitation came from the reconstruction process. They had to detach my pectorals to insert the expander bags, and a lot of the pain came from this. There was severe nerve pain because all the nerve endings had been severed.

I remembered my mother didn't have reconstruction, and she was digging in the garden four days after her surgery. She was told to rest in front of the television for a week or so. She hated television but thought she should give it a go. Mum flicked on the TV and all she saw was violence. She flicked from station to station and found nothing but disturbing images. Mum thought "forget this" and went downstairs to do some gardening. She said that she got tired and couldn't get back up the stairs, so she thought she may as well just stay downstairs and keep gardening—all day. She also told me she had no pain relief after her surgery because she didn't know how to operate the self-administered morphine drip. She had nothing, not even a Panadol. But why am I even comparing myself to her? She is superhuman. She is also crazy. Mum went back to work two weeks after her mastectomy.

She worked in the Special Ed unit at the local Catholic school and turned up there wearing a 44DD bra stuffed with two balloons, saying to her colleagues, "So you thought I was having them off!" They broke the mold when my mum was made.

I was looking forward to going home to start my healing. Apart from the pain and the immobilization of my arms, I was feeling pretty good. It was a dramatic time in my life, and I suppose, being an actor, I have an inherent love of all things dramatic. I received lots of flowers and messages from friends who thought I was so brave. I didn't feel brave, just practical, really, but I breathed in their sympathy and felt rather strong.

15

post-op pain
and impatience

Once home, I realized there was little I could do but rest. Without the use of my arms, there was no housework for me, and I must admit I am a strange fish when it comes to housework: I love it. So I was sure I could read all those books I'd been meaning to. Wrong! I couldn't hold the book up for too long and was too doped out anyway. I just had to breathe through the pain and wait.

Looking back, my little boy was so amazing. I had prepared him for the surgery but had no idea how things would play out during recovery. He came to visit me in the hospital after two days, and I made everything very upbeat for him. He loved the hospital bed that he could manipulate into strange and wonderful positions with the controller. I was so afraid that he would accidentally touch my breasts, but he never once hurt me. It's like there was a force field around my chest when Kaspar was around, and I take no responsibility for that. He created the force field; he was instinctively aware.

At home, he was so gentle with me while still running around like the crazy four-year-old that he was, and this helped me enormously to just get on with it. Kids are good medicine like that: you just can't fall apart, and you have to be the carer no matter how much caring you think you might need. It was not all roses, though, as my recovery went on. I found I had a very short fuse. I became so irritable at times. Kaspar had never really experienced that side of me. If there is one great gift that comes with motherhood, I would say that it is learning patience. Patience is such a precious attribute, and seen as almost archaic in our modern lifestyle. Before motherhood, I never had the opportunity or ability to just stand there and patiently allow a one-year-old to pull every single shoe out of the shoe cupboard with great determination, for the third time. Even the other day, I was folding a huge pile of washing in my bedroom, and Kaspar came in to "help." The chore disintegrated into a fantastic clothes fight, and my bedroom was littered with undies, socks, and jeans. It was fun. I consciously stopped myself from saying, "Don't do that!" And I had the thrill of hearing Kaspar's peals of laughter as we threw one clothes bomb after another at each other. It took me less than five minutes to pick up all the clothes, and I sat and refolded them. However, the one casualty from this surgery was that very same delicate virtue. Pain makes you very cranky, and Kaspar was in the firing line. I hate thinking about it. It must have been a huge thing for a little boy to go through, seeing his mum in so much pain with stitched-on nipples. But children are so resilient and wise, and I have to believe he will simply forget.

I remember one day trying to get Kaspar to put his clothes on when we had to get somewhere. He had other concerns, like fixing up a Lego catastrophe. My pain and patience canceled each other out, and I got cross with him. He protested, "Don't speak to me like that." Now, my mother was there also and in turn yelled at him, "Don't speak to your mother like that." I said, "Mum, just let me deal with it." Interestingly, she replied, "No, you are my daughter, and I won't have you spoken to like that." My mother saw me suffering, and just as I would do anything to protect Kaspar, she was trying to protect me from my own son. All I could do was burst into tears—everyone was unhappy, and I was too sore to fix it.

During those six weeks of recovery, Kaspar said to me many times, "Mummy, you are speaking to me very badly," "Mummy, you are making me very sad," and "Mummy, you are not nice to me." Oh, it broke my heart. The pain was bigger than me, and I couldn't be the mother that I wanted to be. I couldn't hug him, pick him up, or roll around and tickle him because of these stupid breasts that had once fed and nourished him. Another standout nightmare moment was with Sam. The day after I got home, he helped me put on a thin cotton singlet. It was awkward getting it on, and once it was on, I began to panic and yell, "Get it off, get it off!" The weight of this thin little singlet on my chest was unbearable. Sam ran and got the kitchen scissors and cut the thing off in an instant, God bless him. But this is not the nightmare moment.

After the singlet assault, I just lay down without a top on. Sam had already changed my dressings for the day, and he was busy doing the washing and looking after Kaspar. I asked him if he could rub my tummy for a few minutes because he is a really good massage therapist and I was completely backed up, having not been to the toilet in six days. Hospital drugs stop you feeling pain, but they also stop everything from working. At the hospital, they tried to move my bowels with various methods, all unsuccessful. So there was Sam up to his eyeballs in keeping it together, and he said, "I'll rub your tummy if you say thanks for all the hard work I'm doing for you."

I completely flipped out. I have always been very independent and hate having to ask for help. I seethed, "Get out, get out! Here I am with my breasts cut off, completely helpless, and you want me to thank you for cleaning up and looking after your own son! You want me to beg and say please and thank you when I already feel completely humiliated just asking you. We are family, and this is what you do for family. You shouldn't require thanks for just doing what you need to do for your family. GET OUT!"

I was so upset; feeling powerless does not sit well with me. I like to be in control, and this episode made me realize that at that moment, I was completely dependent on those around me. I lay there feeling hideous and vulnerable. In hindsight, I think Sam just wanted me to say, "You're doing okay, mate" because he must have been freaking out too, seeing me in so much pain and not being able to take it away. Oh, hindsight can be so humiliating.

It was a beautiful time in some ways. All the women in my life gathered round with collective empathy. My sisters, my mother, Sam's mother, and some die-hard girlfriends lent their sympathies in practical and spiritual ways. My sister took me to the hairdressers to get my hair washed because I couldn't lift my arms to do it myself. I think she warned them of my condition because they all looked at me with such compassion, imagining themselves prematurely breastless. I never felt pity from other women, just a kind of understated sympathy that I accepted gladly.

I can't say I felt the same around men. Why should I have expected anything? They don't have breasts, so how could they possibly understand the emotional attachment we have to them? Men see breasts in ways that I will never understand. I sensed the men around me just felt it was all a bit gross, just like periods and hemorrhoids during pregnancy. As I walked around with a strange-looking, unnaturally flat torso, I noticed I felt self-conscious and prickly around men in general.

One week after my surgery, I was off to see Dr. D for my post-surgery checkup. He was happy with the wounds and asked if I was ready to start the pumping up. I wasn't prepared for this—I thought it would be further down the track. I was already in so much pain I couldn't imagine any more. But I told myself, he's done this before, and the sooner I start the process the sooner it will be over. Dr. D said it would be uncomfortable afterwards but not too bad.

He pulled out a long needle—I'm talking *long*, as long as a pencil—that sent a shiver of horror down my spine. He ran a magnet over my breasts to find the magnet in my expander bags that housed the entry valve for the saline. He inserted the needle, and because I no longer had sensation in my breast, I couldn't even feel a prick. As the saline went in, my breast inflated right before my eyes. Once again, I felt incredible pressure on my chest, like a couple of sumo wrestlers were sitting there.

When I sat up, I actually had boobs again. He had put in about 150 milliliters. When Dr. D had removed my breast tissue and weighed it, it was 300 grams. So I had half the size of my previous breasts on my first pump-up session. The shape was very strange. The expander bags are quite square and sit up high under the pecs. So it looked like I had big, muscular pectorals similar to that of a male bodybuilder.

The next few days, I paid the price of the pump-up with a new level of pain. The pectorals were angry, as they were being forced to stretch, and the nerve pain was more intense. My sister advised I take pain medication before my next pump-up to preempt the pain. I had gone off all pain meds a week after surgery because they really made me groggy, which is no good when you've got a little one to care for.

Happily, as each day passed, the pain grew less. At my second pump-up, I was prepared with painkillers and in a much better frame of mind. Before he whipped out the needle, I said to Dr. D, "I need to do something before you start because I know I won't be able to do it after," and with that said, I put my hands around his neck and strangled him, just a little. I said, "That's for what you're about to do to me. And by the way, stop lying to your patients, telling them it will feel just a little uncomfortable. It hurts, really hurts."

It was about week four when I emerged from this intensely debilitating state. Everything was progressing well. My scars were healing, the pain was subsiding, and there were bumps that looked vaguely breast-like. When Chrissy was recovering, she went down an emotional hole for a few weeks—the pain wasn't as much an issue for her as the grief was. I would call Chrissy and say, "It's week two, and I haven't started crying yet. When did you start crying?" I was waiting for this emotional response to hit me. It never came.

I didn't feel sad, but I did feel angry. The pain fueled my anger, and the anger fueled my pain. The breast area is so prominent. It's where your heart resides, it is where your hands go to when you are gesticulating passionately, it's the first point of contact when you hug someone, and it is the most obvious reflection of a woman's sensuality. Before my surgery, I protested that my breasts were not that important—certainly not as high a priority as my life—and this is still true, but you don't know what you've got till it's gone.

I don't want to sound like a whiner. People have life-saving surgeries all the time with horrendous recovery periods; but the difference was that my breasts were perfectly healthy when they were removed and may have always stayed that way. The surgery made me understand the intrinsic value of these beautiful, fleshy mounds, and now I would have to find a way to happily live without them.

Around week four after my surgery, I had to attend a cast and crew screening of *Girl Clock*. I was a little nervous about being in a crowd in case anyone bumped my chest. I had been walking around since my surgery with a very protective posture. My shoulders were quite concave and my hands were always clasped together in front of my breasts, like I was in a perpetual state of prayer. But I had little choice but to go, and I took my mother to be my bodyguard. I didn't know what to wear—my boobs looked odd, so a glamorous frock was out of the question. Instead I covered up with a loose jacket buttoned up from my waist to my neck.

My girlfriend Queenie, who was in the film also, was the only one there who knew of my surgery. She was also the only one who elbowed me in the chest more than once while wildly gesticulating. It was pretty funny, really. We watched the film, and I spent most of the movie looking at my former breasts on the screen. Queenie spent most of the film looking at what she thought was her enormous bum. We both complained about the lighting and how it showed all of our wrinkles, although I don't think it was entirely the fault of the lighting. At least I had a permanent record, on celluloid, that I once had a real and naturally undulating bosom. It should have been a big night for me; this was my first important role in a feature film, and everyone was excited about it. But I left as soon as I could.

The best thing about pain is that when it goes, you can hardly even remember it being there in the first place. After week six, I was driving again and trying to get fit for a show I had coming up. If you had spoken to me at this stage, I would have said, "Oh, the surgery was fine—a mere six weeks out of my life to ensure I won't get breast cancer." I'd had just two pump-ups because I only wanted my breasts to be as big as they were before the surgery. There was a four-month wait before the swap-over surgery to give time for the pectorals to expand enough to hold the implants later. In these four months, I had to fit in a show. It was a Force Majeure show called *The Age I'm In*, which I had done before and which was being revived for two weeks at the Carriageworks in Sydney.

I had to get my fitness up because it was a physical theater show. During rehearsals, we had to change a few things to accommodate my situation. I could no longer do a scene that involved lifting, carrying, and throwing a young man around. I also couldn't hold my own body weight up with my arms; my pectorals just didn't seem to work. But I tried to do push-ups each day, and it increased my strength. This was hilarious for me, just privately, because when I engaged my pec muscle, it lifted the whole boob up. Normally the pectoral is behind the breast tissue, but now it was the breast tissue, so when my pec moved, my boobs moved. I was having a problem viewing my boobs as boobs. At this stage, as far as I was concerned, I didn't have "boobs" any longer. I had strange bags under my pecs that were filled with water. They didn't feel like boobs, not by a long shot, and they hardly looked like boobs. But I had to refer to them as something.

My female colleagues wanted to have a good look. I was happy to show them and get it out of the way so I wouldn't feel weird in the dressing room. They marveled at the smallness of the scars across my nipples, thanks to the clever Dr. D, whom I only strangled once. I made them feel the metal magnets under my skin, and that freaked them out a little. Also, the expander bags have this half moon of hard plastic, like Tupperware plastic, and feeling that made the ladies cringe. Breasts are meant to feel soft and supple and, as any woman knows, they are very sensitive, especially around menstruation time. The idea of having plastic and metal in there made all the ladies look a little green around the gills.

During this time, I was actually quite shameless

about showing my bosom. Anyone who was curious got a look. It didn't feel rude because they didn't feel like mine. I wasn't showing people my breasts; I was showing them some weird science experiment that was happening on my chest. Perhaps it was a way of helping me to accept what was going on—self-therapy, sharing the burden around. Only once it backfired when I met up with a long-time girlfriend of mine who nearly gagged when I showed her. She said, "No, no please don't; that's horrible." I don't blame her at all. It's not very fair to thrust people into an uncomfortable position and expect them to respond in a positive way.

I kept touching them also. My hands would just go there unconsciously, shifting things around because it was uncomfortable or because of a sudden sharp pain. It was a little disconcerting in public for people to see me seemingly fondling my own boobs. Sam would say, "You're always touching them."

The show was relatively easy to execute with my makeshift chest. The expander bags were extremely uncomfortable but not painful.

The afternoon before our opening night, one of the cast members, Roz, became injured. She was one of the dancers, and all eyes looked to me to take over all of her scenes. For about three hours, we rehearsed madly as I tried to learn all of her choreography. It was quite sur-real as we negotiated moves that could, under the circum-stances, risk a breast explosion. I danced, flipped, and threw myself around, but luckily Roz went on with the aid of last-minute treatments and painkillers. The show must go on. No matter if you are sick, dying, or even deceased, shows will never be canceled. I have performed with a bucket side stage so I could run off and vomit during a scene. Any normal job would allow a person to stay home if at death's door.

I was booked in to have my swap-over surgery two days before Christmas 2008. I couldn't wait. I just wanted it all to be over so I could get on with my life without my breasts being the complete focus of every minute of every day. I was over talking about them, touching them, complaining about them, eliciting sympathy for them, and making everybody look at them. Who cares? Put them away! It's just a bit of breast tissue; they just removed some tissue from my body! Why then was it such a big deal? Why is it that that particular bodily tissue seems to represent my womanhood? I didn't have any answers to this conundrum at this stage, but the random, searing nerve pain that momentarily took my breath away kept me asking the questions.

16

swap-over

surgery

I was so ready for my swap-over surgery. The expanders were ugly and uncomfortable. I never thought I would be looking forward to getting silicone implants, but there I was, prepped and ready for my "boob job."

Dr. D had shown me the implant options available. There was the question of size, of course. Friends and family had varying opinions about what size I should have. Most everybody said to go bigger. However, I steadfastly wanted implants as close to the size of my original breasts as possible. Bigger is not necessarily better, in my opinion. I was very concerned about looking like someone who'd had a breast "enhancement." "Enhance" means to intensify, to magnify; I just wanted to replace what was taken away.

There was a profusion of shapes to choose from. I could feel Great-Grandma Maude and Grandma Elsie looking over my shoulder again with eyebrows raised. Seriously, there were hundreds of breast shapes: high profile, low profile, teardrop, and every imaginable variation. I just said I want a small, natural-looking breast. Dr. D chose one, and I trusted him.

This second surgery was a breeze compared to the first. Dr. D made the incisions through my nipples again. With Chrissy's second surgery, she had incisions made under the breast, as her nipples were a no-go zone. One of the risks with this nipple-preserving mastectomy is necrosis of the nipple. The surgeon has the delicate job of removing as much tissue as possible while leaving a sustainable blood supply to keep the nipple alive. A week after Chrissy's mastectomy, she watched in horror as one of her nipples turned black. She was scratching at it, and the tip of it fell off. It is really not very noticeable: she only lost about one-third of her nipple in the end.

My nipples had survived brilliantly and were ready to be put under the knife again. In the operating room, Dr. D said, "I have your implants here, and I brought a bigger size as well." What a bloke—bigger, bigger, bigger, more, more, more! "I'll have the smaller ones, please," I said with a smile and then slipped into that most unnatural of sleeps.

When I awoke, the first thing I saw was my mother. At any daunting moment in my life, I have opened my eyes to see my mother there, simply sitting, quietly composed. I immediately opened my surgical bra with the coordination of a drunkard, and I was happy. My breasts were soft and supple again; they weren't square, and they were brilliant. Mum whipped out the camera, which was never far from her reach.

I was relieved it was all finished, and I was so grateful that I could have a life-saving surgery and then the added privilege of an amazing reconstruction. I saw Maude and Elsie nodding and smiling to each other in wonderment.

I went home from the hospital on Christmas Eve, doped out and emotional from the drugs. When coming out of general anesthetic, you are on a mini emotional roller coaster. The world was getting drunk and singing stupid songs, and I was ducking off to the toilet to have a little sob. I was not at all feeling sorry for myself or unhappy about my breasts, just getting toxins out of my body through streams of tears.

On Christmas Day, our family had organized to have a homeless luncheon. We hired a hall and attempted to feed one hundred homeless and disadvantaged people in our area. It was a great day. We had collected so many gifts to give away and everyone had a hot three-course Christmas meal. We had almost as many volunteers as homeless people, so all our guests were made to feel very special indeed. Sam entertained the masses, singing a myriad of Christmas carols dressed as Santa in shorts and thongs.

All I could manage to do was sit on the steps of the stage and blow bubbles from one of those kiddie bubble bottles. At one stage, Chrissy said to a volunteer, "There's a lady on table one who seems all alone; could you go keep her company?" The volunteer pointed to me and said, "Do you mean that lady there who looks like she is on drugs?" Chrissy said, "No, that's just my sister."

In the parking lot after the luncheon, our family exchanged gifts. We had decided to have a recycled Christmas. You could only give a gift that was home-made or secondhand, and wrapped in recycled Christmas paper. I received a dress from Chrissy that she had stolen from me twenty years ago. I had all but forgotten about it. She'd had it repaired and dry-cleaned. Elisha gave me a pair of groovy jeans of hers that I had been eyeing for a long time. There were other gifts, such as an out-of-date bottle of salad dressing and a half-eaten chocolate bar. It was a great way to palm off all those gifts you had received in previous years that never saw the light of day. We gathered up all the paper to be used again and went home satisfied that our Christmas was the opposite of consumer frenzy. They didn't fit the recycled theme, but I was more than content with my pair of fake breasts for Christmas.

I had four weeks to recover before starting rehearsals on a new show. Once the drugs wore off, there was little to recover from. I wore a surgical bra 24/7 and changed the dressings on my nipples weekly. It was more about getting to know my new boobs. I kept feeling them, looking at them, and trying on all my clothes to see how they fit. They were slightly bigger, but really quite modest. I was stoked that they were small enough not to be mistaken for a boob job. Nobody in their right mind would pay for a boob job this small.

Finally I could sleep on my side again. I had been sleeping on my back since my first surgery, always aware not to roll over. Kaspar jumps into my bed at about three every morning, and I was terrified that he would kick or whack me in his sleep. He seriously turns into a donkey come nightfall. I even wore bumper bars on my arms that the breast cancer nurse gave me. They were U-shaped pillows you slip up over your arms to protect you from accidental blows to the boobs. But, of course, my brilliant boy never so much as grazed me. It was a sexy time, I can assure you—I was terrifically lucky to be single.

All the pain and awkwardness had gone with the expanders. All that was left was some lingering nerve pain in my left nipple that hurt when fabric rubbed against it, and occasional sharp jabs out of nowhere. Christine is about a year ahead of me, and she testifies that every day brings improvement.

Even though there was no general pain anymore, a very strange thing was happening. Sometimes I would feel a shooting pain; my hand would instinctively touch my breast, and at that instant, tears would well in my eyes. I have no idea why. There seemed to be no corresponding feeling of anguish—there was no thought at all; just an overwhelming moment of despair. This would happen at least once a day and continues to happen to this day. Psychologists would have a field day with this, I'm sure, but I don't want to unravel it. I just want to allow it to happen and sit in it. As fleeting as it is, it is both sad and beautiful.

17

getting to know

the new *(pieces of)* me

After my reconstruction, it took some time to get to know my new breasts and adjust my brain to my new body. My name, Veronica, means "true image." Veronica was a biblical character who wiped the face of Jesus as he carried his cross towards crucifixion. On the cloth that she'd used, there appeared the face of Jesus. A "true image" of Christ, captured for all time, on her humble hanky. Now, I know Jesus's face has turned up on pizzas and various bits of fruit and vegetables since, but Veronica's cloth was the first.

I'm wondering what a true image is. Whether I am looking at myself or someone else is looking at me, the image is distorted by subjectivity. I can't look to external sources for guidance on what is true and not true. Throughout history we have conformed to arbitrary standards of the human image that seem to change with the wind. All I know is that my image is altered. I need not compare it to what is accepted or fashionable—I just need to realign myself with it.

I feel different when I look at myself, but I also feel different when I am not looking at myself. Before I had my mastectomy, I could always feel my breasts. I don't mean with my hands, but intrinsically. Just as an amputee can still feel their lost limb, I can still sense my breasts, but it doesn't feel quite the same. They feel like impostors. As time goes on, I may reconcile myself to this fact or maybe the impostors will have dissolved the memory of my real breasts and I will unwittingly forget.

I am not complaining. These new breasts are disease-free, they are pert, they are firm. But when my arm bumps against them, it feels as if I have bumped into someone else. I feel like saying, "Oh, excuse me," and then I realize it's just me.

They are numb. I have a sense of weight, but that's about it. Chrissy said that sometimes after she's been on the phone at work, she'll look at her computer screen and see lines of random letters and spaces. She has not been aware that her boobs have been typing away without her knowledge. The numbness is a strange mix of a deadened feeling and nerve spasm. It feels a bit like the sensation you get when a dental anesthetic is just beginning to wear off—your face feels dead to the touch but a little tingly. I hate it when one of my breast pretends to be itchy; I scratch and scratch away at numb skin to no avail. Some-where deep down in my subconscious there is the echo of an itch that will never be scratched.

They are cold. Because I have no breast tissue, the implant is really only covered with a thin layer of skin.

When it's winter, my boobs are like two little ice packs. They don't make me feel cold, but if I touch them, my hand retracts with the chill. My sister and I have been discussing the need for someone to invent an "ugg bra" for those with breast reconstructions, or a thermal inlay that heats up when the skin on the breast drops below zero. I know what to do now when I burn my hand on the stove—shove it straight in my bra.

Memory can be a bit of a shape shifter, I know, but I seem to remember that I had beautiful breasts. Oh, they were not outrageously voluptuous or even perfect but they were beautiful. I never spent any time assessing them as such; I just felt that they were. I am not ready to throw open my shirt right now. It so happens that there is no invitation for me to do so at present, but I am glad of that. I would feel insecure and uncomfortable with them being looked upon as a thing of pleasure. I think I will need to grow to love them before I can expect anyone else to.

My breasts are many things, but mainly they are maternal and sexual. As it stands, their maternal role is over and done with and their sexual future remains a mystery. Chrissy had a great deal of trepidation about having her breasts removed because they played a huge role in her sexual relationship with her husband, Ray. They were so sensitive that she needed little more than a touch to drive her to the peak of pleasure; this in turn gave Ray all the satisfaction in the world because he was behind that wheel. Now, because Chrissy has no sensation in her breasts at all, they both are at a bit of a loss as to what to do with them in the bedroom. Ray has said he thinks they look great but because Chrissy can't feel them, he is not that interested in touching them. She complained to me the other day that when they have sex now she just keeps her shirt on. There is a veritable standoff in the bedroom with Chrissy and Ray on one side and her new boobs on the other. It leaves her wondering now what she got them for.

Whether I like it or not, my body is part of my social existence. Having a reconstruction makes me feel more comfortable in public—it's so much easier than having to explain to people why I have no breasts at my age. My mother is totally okay with her body image. She wears her scars proudly and was always whipping her prosthesis out at any provocation, before she skewered it with the pitchfork. Chrissy told me once that she and Ray held a Lindy Hop dance and hired a band to play. The numbers were low and they had not taken enough cash at the door to pay the band. My mother decided to whip out her prosthesis and charge people five dollars to have a photo taken with it. I think they only made thirty dollars from this racket, but it shows the shamelessness of my mum in terms of vanity or social expectation.

My mother was the one who suggested that I could cope with having no reconstruction. Ultimately it is safer not to reconstruct because more breast tissue can be removed and it is easier to detect changes to the breast area in the future. Sometimes I imagine myself having no reconstruction. I think I would have come to terms with it in the long run. It would have been more difficult psychologically, for sure, but I always speculate that it would have been a braver choice for me. I would have been able to challenge the stereotypes of beauty in society and discover where my own true beauty lies beyond my physical appearance. Would've, should've, could've. I will never know.

Let's face it, I am no Saint Agatha. Saint Agatha of Sicily was persecuted for her Christian faith in the third century. A Roman judge had taken a liking to her, and when she refused his amorous advances, he sent her to a brothel, tortured her, and cut off her breasts. She was later sentenced to death at the stake, but a mysterious earthquake shook the ground, and the burning was canceled. She died in prison soon after. Depictions of Saint Agatha show her carrying her breasts around on a plate. She is the patron saint of breast cancer. Perhaps when I am struggling with self-pity I will call to mind Agatha's peril and pull my head in.

18

back *to* work

Four weeks after my swap-over surgery, I was back to
work with my new boobs, and all was good. I didn't
have any bras to wear because all my old ones no longer
fit. I still measured the same in my chest (91 centimeters,
or 36 inches) but I was now a C cup instead of a B cup.
They were still settling down, and it would probably be
another three months before I would know their true size.
I was as poor as a church mouse after maxing out my
credit card on my surgeries, so new bras had to wait. I
just wore old T-shirt bras that had no underwiring and
were a bit too small.

I was in a new show called *White Earth*. It was an
adaptation of an Australian novel written by Andrew
McGahan. The show was going to be performed at the
La Boite Theatre Company in Brisbane and was a play
that only required me to walk and talk and not bump into

the furniture. In other words, it was not a physical theatre show where I could sustain injury. My breasts debuted nicely, and those who knew of my surgeries were very impressed with their performance. On opening night, I took the opportunity to wear a top that showed them off nicely, and I was heard to proclaim proudly, more than once, "What mastectomy?"

One thing people may not know about actors is that there is a collective unconscious when it comes to nightmares. As young children we all have nightmares about showing up at school in our pajamas or without pants or with ridiculous bunny slippers on. Kaspar had his first one the other day. I was dressing him for school and he said, "I have got my pants on, haven't I?" I said, "Yes, of course, darling," and he told me he'd had the nightmare. So this is an actor's nightmare: we find ourselves on stage in a play that we don't know and cannot remember rehearsing. We race backstage to look for a script, and every copy that we find is either in another language or has had the required scenes ripped out of them. Some variations of this nightmare are hearing your cue to go on but not being able to find the stage, or you are unable to find your costume and are completely naked.

Usually about a week before a new show is about to open, I start having these dreams, and it's a good reminder that things are right on track.

Some of the more tangible daily fears for actors are, of course, forgetting your lines in front of an audience (drying), or simply falling flat on your face, literally. Well, I am here to say that after twenty years of sure-footedly treading the boards, it finally happened to me. A few weeks after opening, I was running on to make a dramatic entrance, and I tripped on one of the floor lights and landed completely prostrate in front of around four hundred strangers. I was face down, arms completely outstretched, as if in abject prayer. There was no way to recover cleverly, this was not a comedy, and it was obvious that it wasn't meant to happen. So I simply chose to ignore it, got up, and continued the scene. After the curtain call, I raced off, locked myself in the toilets, and sobbed.

Firstly, I have never felt more humiliated, and secondly, it scared me because I landed right on my newly reconstructed breasts. I was crying and grabbing at them to feel if I had burst them or split open the wounds. They didn't hurt because they were numb, but I had been protecting them with my life for the last six months, and this was a full-frontal blow. It was like a dam had burst; I sat on the loo and cried and cried. I realized that there was so much emotion trapped in there and it was good to be releasing some of it. I think it was a good thing to happen to me as an actor too because I had passed through one of my worst fears and could now cross it off the list. I had to eventually come out of the toilet because I was sharing the dressing room with three other ladies. I came out all red-eyed and puffy. They asked, "What's up?" I told them I'd fallen flat on my face, and it turned out they hadn't even noticed.

At the end of that season, I went straight into rehearsal for a new show with the Queensland Theatre Company, *God of Carnage* by Yasmina Reza. I was playing the role of Veronique Vallon, and it was a great role. This play was the hot new ticket around the world; it was a hit on the West End and Broadway, with famous actors in the casts. People kept asking if I felt intimidated by the thought that

Marcia Gay Harden and Isabelle Huppert had played the role of Veronique. I wasn't. I was unaware of any previous productions, for one, but also, as an actor cast in this role, I had every chance of doing just as good a job as another actor, whether they were famous or not. Fame does not necessarily equal talent.

When I tell people that I'm an actor, I find it curious when they ask, "Are you famous? Have you been in any movies or TV shows?" Well, I have. I've been working nonstop for twenty years and have worked on dozens of films and television programs, but I am not famous. I am simply and proudly a jobbing actor. The general public thinks that success in our industry is measured by how famous you are. For those of us who are actors, success is weighed with very different scales. There are thousands of actors working in Australia—talented, skilled, and with great bodies of work behind them—who are not famous but are continually employed because they are good at their job.

Let's face it, there can only be a handful of famous actors at any one time, and they need to be surrounded by a bunch of other actors from which to stand out. I am one of those other actors, just beavering away at my job. I like to see myself as a public servant, really. The arts are an intrinsic part of our social fabric, a public platform for political and social debate, and are still largely funded by the government. So I work for the government, channeling the ideas of writers who are helping the public to better understand the nature of our humanity. My job description is to tell the story, not to be famous. That's what I am going to say next time someone says, "Have I seen ya on the telly?"

There are exceptions. I do think some people were born under very favorable stars: Geoffrey Rush, Cate Blanchett, Fiona Shaw, Daniel Day Lewis, to name a few. But these people are just geniuses, not to be compared with us mere mortals in any way. If the likes of Cate or Fiona had played Veronique Vallon before me, I would be intimidated—I would poop my pants.

During rehearsal, I began to notice that one of my breast implants was behaving strangely. Dr. D told me that he would need to stitch my implants in at the sides to help keep them in place. After a mastectomy and without breast tissue, the implants are held in place with only the pectoral muscle, so some added stitching can help. However, there is very little to hold the stitches because all the breast tissue is gone and I don't have a lot of excess fat in that area. So it seemed one of my implants had walked right on through the stitching and was heading in the direction of my back.

I went to see Dr. D and said I really didn't think I wanted a back boob and could he fix it up. He tried to sell my "back boob" to me as a party trick. He had done this before: when I showed how my whole implants lifted up when engaging my pec he called it a "party trick." Well, I don't know what parties Dr. D indulges in, but I said, "No, not a party trick this time." Of course he could fix it—he could go in there and restitch it for me. But it would mean a new scar under my breast and another general anesthetic. He did not want to risk going in through my nipples again because they seemed very healthy and they had been removed twice already.

I was bummed. I thought it could just be a keyhole job through the armpit. I didn't want another surgery.

But we scheduled it in for two weeks after *God of Carnage* finished. While filling out the paperwork, he slyly asked, "Happy with your size, are you?" with the sort of rising inflection that has a certain presumption about it. I told him I was more than happy with the size. He said, "Well, when your implants need replacing in ten or so years, you can maybe upgrade." Incorrigible!

I upgraded to a new bra, though. It was a hand-me-down maternity bra from my brother's partner, Sharon. Dr. D had told me that it would take a few months after the swap-over surgery, when all the swelling had settled, to work out exactly what size I was. It was four months now, and Sharon's bra fit like a treat. I was a 12C! I didn't know this before, but finding out what bra size you are helps with your sense of identity. "Hello, my name is Veronica Neave, and I am a 12C."

The show was a hit, and I loved playing Veronique Vallon. I looked hot with my new bra, and nobody ever suspected I had a fake front boob that wanted to be a back boob. I was ready for my third surgery, but with growing trepidation. I began to be confronted with my own expectations from this reconstruction. I did need to secure this implant again because as time went on, it didn't seem to stop sliding, and it was uncomfortable as it forged new ground. But I needed to keep in mind the reality that this was a reconstruction and I was never going to have a perfect set of breasts. I did hope that this would be my last surgery and that I could accept my breasts and their peculiarities and just get on with it.

I have to keep reminding myself that my sister and I have had reconstructive surgery and need to be realistic about how our breasts look and feel now. I found the

FORCE website to be a useful resource and a great support group and online community set up to help people affected by hereditary breast and ovarian cancer. Many stories on the FORCE website tell of women who are elated with their new breasts, which I think is a bonus outcome for a lifesaving surgery. I love reading the stories of the women who chose not to reconstruct and feel so liberated because they are now flat-chested. There is part of me that wonders how I would feel if I had gone that way: less pain, fewer surgeries, fewer bikini tops. Mostly I identify with many of the women over forty who feel slightly ridiculous having such pert breasts at a mature age. However, there are some women who may never come to terms with the loss of their natural breasts, and their reconstructed breasts may never look right.

19

hoping *for a* happy ending

It's July 2009—nearly a year since I had my breasts removed—and here I am again, facing Dr. de Viana in my paper hat and paper undies, hopefully for the last time. He draws all over my breast with his little marker and takes some ever-so-glamorous photos. He always looks cute in his surgical blues, and I am not anxious at all about the outcome; he's a master boob man.

I tell Dr. D that I am almost finished with my book and that whether the book has a happy ending or a tragic one all depends on him. He promises to give me a happy ending. I sleep the sleep once more. I wake in my hospital room a little disappointed because I paid for a private room but there were only shared rooms available. I'm alone for about six hours, though. I have a self-administered pain-relief drip, but the more I push the button, the more I get a headache. The thrill of the hospital drugs is over.

The thrill of this whole journey is over. I am so relieved to be having my last surgery so I can just get on with life and not be at the mercy of the machinations of my chest. I think those around me are over it too. The night before my surgery, Sam and Kaspar left to stay at Kaspar's grandparents' house. Sam forgot to even say good luck for my surgery. My parents were away; they had driven across the Nullarbor in their campervan to visit Loo Loo. But Chrissy was there, of course, to drop me off.

Some hours later, they wheel in my roommate, Alice. Through the curtains, I hear feeble moans, slurred words, and then the telltale sentence: "It feels like there are elephants sitting on my chest." Poor Alice. At that moment, I realize how far I have come; I am an old hand. Alice is right at the beginning of this horrendous trial—she is me one year ago. I want to hug her right away and say how brave she is and that there will be an end, but I am all wired up, so I just lie there feeling her anxiety and loneliness through the partition.

I muse on the future of the BRCA2-Neave connection. I wonder where it will end. My mother still needs to be vigilant, having had breast cancer twice and with one breast remaining on her chest. They won't remove her other breast because the Warfarin she takes for her heart makes surgery too risky. Chrissy and I too will need to be aware that a cancer could still appear, though the risks are slight.

Chrissy's friend Sue is recovering and seems to be in a good place now. She was thrown into menopause from the chemotherapy. If the chemo didn't do it, the hysterectomy would have. I can only imagine how much her body has had to endure with the cancer, mastectomy, reconstruction, chemo, and hysterectomy all piling on top of each other. Then, of course, to process all of this emotionally must have been overwhelming, to say the least. She is healthy again and feels that she has really made a difference for her family in uncovering the BRCA2 gene. It is information that she feels her family can use in a proactive way if they so choose in the future.

Her boys are not yet grown up, but she feels she has given them a choice to investigate this mutation if they have daughters. Her sister is certainly happy that Sue's discovery has allowed her to prevent the possibility of ovarian cancer.

One of Sue's big concerns is getting a tumor behind her implants. The very fact that you can get breast cancer even after a mastectomy is just salt to the wound, really. It is a low-risk scenario, but it happened to my mum, so it's in my mind. I will try not to worry too much about it, though, because at some point I feel as though I have to say, "What will be will be." I cannot control everything. Chrissy and I both need to consider removing our ovaries before too long since ovarian cancer is hard to detect under surveillance. But for now, I just want to forget about it and dig my head in the sand a little until my scars heal.

I drift in and out and think of little Ziggi, my only niece. My brother Denny, her father, has not had the gene test as yet. If he does and tests positive, Ziggi can decide if she wants to be tested when she is eighteen years old. By that time, it will be the year 2025, and hopefully the medicine will have caught up with the science. In Ziggi's time, they may be able to switch the BRCA2 gene off altogether with a little pill, or at the very least grow her brand new breasts from stem cells. Whatever science fiction plays out, Ziggi is sure to look back on her old Auntie Ronnie as a survivor of macabre practices. "Back in the old days," she will say, "can you believe they used to chop women's healthy breasts off?" I will have embellished the story by then for sure, adding, "Yes, and they did it with no anesthetic, and I had to help the surgeon by holding my nipples for him till he sewed them back on!"

I overhear a phone call Alice is making to her family. She is reassuring them that she is just fine. I realize she has a small child because I hear her say, "No, Mummy's boobs are gone now. Yes, they're not there any more, darling." Throughout the night, the nurse, a sprightly little angel called Michelle, pops in and out, asking her how her pain is, and she says, "It's terribly painful when I move. I feel like it's hard to breathe." There is still a drawn curtain between us, but I hope I get a chance to see her face-to-face before I check out.

There is something very dreamlike about the hospital—apart from the drugs and surgeries. I have found it interesting having a window into this surreal world. There is no night or day; the nurses buzz about around the clock, and you're woken every hour or two for observations. The drugs give you sporadic sleep and unnatural dreams. You just don't know when you're actually awake or asleep—you don't quite feel like you're on Earth anymore. I open my eyes and catch a glimpse of an old man shuffling past my room, not sure if I am dreaming or if he is Dad walking past my door.

My dad is going through a renaissance right now. It is so wonderful to see, and a long time coming for him. He is smelling the roses and calling his kids and telling us he loves us. He even sent me flowers on opening night of *God of Carnage* with a note saying he is proud of me and loves me; he has never done that before. He called Chrissy recently and asked her to come over after work just to give him a hug. Mum found him in the garden the other day just marvelling at how beautiful the buffalo grass was. His behavior seems somewhat crazy, but we are loving it. Here is a man who found it painful to communicate for most of his life, and now he calls me to say, "I'm just going to be switching my mobile off for an hour or so, so if you want to reach me, you'll have to wait a bit." I think we had all given up hope that he would come out of his terrible fog, but he has. He cries, he laughs, he is free, and it is nice to have him back. I smile to myself, and the thought of him comforts me as I drift off.

I am awoken from a tormented and furry sleep to see a strange lady opening my hospital gown. "Who are you?" I ask. "I'm Betty. Just looking at your boob." "Ah, Betty the boob lady," I acknowledge, although I have never seen her before. My left breast, which Dr. D operated on, is as swollen as a football. Betty the boob lady is satisfied that I will make it through the night and leaves as mysteriously as she came.

Dr. D comes to see me postsurgery. It's about 10 p.m., and he is still here. I say to him, "What are you still doing here? What about your wife, your kids?" "I know," he says, "I think I have forgotten where I live." He works so hard, and it's such important work too. I feel for his family but am so grateful for the time he has given me. I ask him how many stitches he put in me, but he won't tell me. I think I know why—it feels like there are hundreds. He tells me not to drive for at least a week and to really take it easy for one month. I had factored this in and had left six weeks free before my next job. I will see him at his clinic in one week.

In the morning, I finally chat with Alice. She had found a small cancer in her breast, and because of her history, she wanted them to take everything. She does not know if she has the gene but suspects it is the case. I ask her if she thinks she'll have the gene test, and she tells me that her grown children are not sure if they want to be put in the position of knowing they have a fifty-fifty chance of inheriting it. For Alice the gene test is not really relevant; she has already had a hysterectomy, and now that her breasts have been removed, there is little more she can do. She has a small child too, a little girl, who said to her, "Mummy, you should get your DNA tested." It's a sign of the times.

Alice looks so vulnerable lying there without her breasts. I decide to take off my shirt and show her what they could look like in one year's time. She is shocked and excited, saying, "Wow, I would love to have breasts that looked like that." Dr. D is her surgeon, so I say, "Well, you probably will." She writes down the implant size that I have because she thinks that it would be perfect for her. I feel happy that I have offered her a little glimpse into the future and it made her less afraid.

Alice and I then rail at the insidiousness of breast cancer. She says, "It seems every woman I talk to lately has breast cancer." Her sister survived it, her aunties all had it. We wonder together why it has to be our breasts— why do our beautiful breasts turn against us? But we both know it's just rhetoric and in the end we are lucky that we are strong enough to put up a fight. I wish Alice all the best of luck and leave the hospital.

20

musings *about* mutations

I've never been one to embrace the old adage "ignorance is bliss," but I am beginning to understand its true value. At an early age, I threw off Catholicism because my questions could no longer find satisfactory answers from rusty old parables. Blind faith was definitely not for me.

One passage from the Bible that did stick with me, though, was St. Paul's letter to the Corinthians: "When I was a child I spake as a child, I understood as a child, I thought like a child; but when I became a man I put aside childish things. For now we see through a glass darkly."

It's not that I'm a pessimist by any means—I just love to embrace reality, deal with the facts, and draw strength from truth and understanding. Knowledge is a gift; I think it is one of the greatest gifts of all. I have always devoured it, dissected it, and even manipulated it into works of art. Yet my experience with BRCA2 has left me wondering if it's true that we can have too much knowledge.

As I see it, information leads to knowledge, which in turn leads to wisdom. The gene identification discoveries provide us with information. With this information, I was able to search out all the knowledge available to me, but I have not yet come close to a place of wisdom. It is all still shrouded in too much mystery. Who can ever tell if I made the right decision? It was simply an educated guess, not a truly wise decision. Technology is pushing ahead at such a rate that most people clearly don't know what to do with the information.

We are living in an era in which our concepts about ourselves are rapidly changing. New understandings of genetics can now shed light on how we're formed, who we may become, and the illnesses that might afflict us. This new knowledge will also have significant ramifications for the community at large.

All of humanity is one family. We can trace our genetic lineages and our roots; we share a common genetic origin. This drives me to ask the question: to what extent should this knowledge be controlled? Should it be used for the benefit of just a few individuals or for the benefit of everyone? If someone is found to have a gene mutation, they may be seen as an anomaly. The mutation may place them "apart" from society or members of their family. But we all carry mutations—we just don't know what they are. What is unusual about someone who carries an identified mutation is not the mutation, but the fact that it is identified. We all have gene mutations, it's just what that gene mutation means in regards to our future physical health—the probability of it becoming a reality that impacts our future. Maybe we shouldn't even use words like faulty genes or mutations; they're such unpleasant labels. How about we just take the bull by the horns and say it: everyone's a mutant.

I am happy with the decisions I've made. I have no regrets, and I feel so grateful that my life may have been saved. But it has made me wonder about the ethical boundaries surrounding predictive gene testing. I've learned recently that in the United States people are having "spit parties," where you can purchase a kit, spit into a tube, send it to a lab, and then, four to six weeks later, explore your genome on the web.

A company called 23andMe, which provides genetic testing for over one hundred traits and diseases as well as DNA ancestry, was voted *Time* magazine's invention of the year in 2008. The company's name is a reference to the twenty-three pairs of chromosomes that contain our DNA. The results of the genetic testing are not actually diagnostic but simply provide you with your particular information.

This information may empower people to take precautions and change detrimental habits to lower their risk percentages. It is really the beginning of an era of customizing care. This could save governments a lot of money by tailoring health care to target specific problems. It could save lives. People could have more power to manage their specific needs and optimize outcomes, turning chance into choice. Ultimately we could live healthier and longer lives.

This ideal of living a ridiculously long and relatively healthy life is still a way off though. Most diseases do not have a clearly defined single genetic component. In fact, around 95 percent of diseases have a complex interplay of

several genes. The BRCA2 gene is a monogenetic mutation, making it easy to point to a likelihood of breast
cancer. But there are millions of diseases that are multi-
genetic in their makeup. Scientists are sweating away,
trying to understand the molecular basis of disease; however, it's still largely unknown as to how it truly trans-
lates into personalized predictions.

There is an enormous amount of genetic information
captured in the genetic code. We can decipher it now, but
does that necessarily mean we should? Perhaps if there's
a good reason for accessing it, we should. We need to
recognize the potential—whether it can be useful or of
benefit—but also that it's not the only thing that shapes
us. Genetics has a key role to play in who we are and who
we will become, but it's not the only factor. So, like most
things, genetics is a very good servant; but do we want to
have it as a master?

It's only in the last decade or so that scientists have
begun to recognize that the environment can change how
the genetic code actually works. Scientists have suspected
for around fifty years that there has to be some mecha-
nism for switching genes on and off, for regulating how
they work. They also know that certain genes can be
switched off for the long term, and this is due to a chemi-
cal change to the gene (methylation). The food we eat can
have some impact on methylation, otherwise known as
gene silencing.

This whole understanding of how genes and the environment interact is still very much in its infancy. Also
in its infancy is the idea of genes interacting with genes.
All of these genes are working together—there are about
twenty-five thousand different genes in each cell, and

there are a million billion cells in each individual. So we can't really relate the behavior of a single cell or a single individual to one particular gene or to one particular environmental influence.

When science does get better at predicting disease susceptibility, there will surely follow a minefield of prejudices and insurance problems. There may be things we find out that will mark us as an undesirable candidate for procreation. When I was pregnant with Kaspar, I remarked on more than one occasion that I had "dipped into a good gene pool" with Sam. He is handsome, athletic, physically strong, and remarkably healthy—what one would call a "good specimen." This has always been a natural and somewhat unconscious aspect to human coupling anyway, but the possibility of picking and choosing from gene pools in a catalogue doesn't sound very sexy.

Should love prevail in spite of genetic incompatibility, there will always be the possibility of having your fetus genotyped or sequenced at birth to iron out any inconvenient gene traits. Designer babies could see our future populated with freckle-less, blue-eyed, slender children with special aptitudes for sports and leadership. On the positive side of this is the opportunity for unborn babies to avoid a life of pain and suffering if an unexpected gene fault is detected and silenced. The nuchal fold test that shows a marker for the possibility of Down syndrome has been around for decades and did provide me with a great sense of relief when I obtained my results.

In the United Kingdom, a couple going through IVF treatment in order to conceive knew that they were carriers of a breast cancer gene. They were able to select an embryo for implantation that did not contain the gene mutation. I could have benefited from this situation: no prophylactic mastectomy, no reconstruction, no need to be contemplating a hysterectomy and oophorectomy. However, if you've seen the futuristic movie *Gattaca*, you'll have some idea of what can happen when genetic engineering is taken to the extreme.

Insurance is such a nightmare already in our society, and the more knowledge an insurance company has, the less likely they are to protect you. I live in a place surrounded by trees, and I'm sure before too long it will be impossible to afford fire insurance. Will insurance companies be able to have access to our dirty genetic secrets? Will only the very rich be able to afford health insurance for preexisting gene faults? The gap between rich and poor may widen further with the affordability of preventive medicine; we could see the creation of a genetic underclass.

The psychological effects of knowing your genetic potentialities is fraught with emotion. Imagine finding out you have a propensity for a certain disease that scares the heck out of you, and you live your life with a feeling of impending doom. Your fear may drive you away from directions you would otherwise have ventured toward, in turn missing opportunities that would have presented themselves along the avoided path. It could make you more pessimistic than you naturally may have been. It could stop you from taking up a particular sport or career for fear of inciting your genetic predisposition. On the other hand, a positive genetic identification could give you a bravado you never knew you had or bring with it a certain complacency that would make you less likely to make healthy lifestyle choices.

That's not all. There is the hot debate about genes and patenting. About five thousand of the twenty-five thousand genes have been patented. That means they are owned by certain parties who proved that they "invented" the genes. Until twenty years ago, an organism—anything that was a product of nature or a law of nature—could not be patented. Gold was discovered, but it could not be patented. A patent is permitted if there is proof of an invention. Those who have patented genes to date could prove they invented the gene because it was isolated from the body; it was taken out of the body and stripped out of its cell.

The BRCA2 gene has been patented. It is owned by Myriad Genetics, which claimed to have isolated the gene. Myriad owns the entire gene and the proteins those genes express. The company controls the information about the gene and decides where to channel the research. Those who argue for patenting contend that it encourages research and investment. Companies that find and isolate genes have put a lot of money into the invention and have rights to make returns on this investment. The whole idea behind patenting is to stimulate innovation.

Opponents argue that patenting inhibits research, that it gives the inventor the monopoly and does not allow broader scientific investigation.

Treating genetic disease is big business, and, as you can imagine, it will get ever bigger. Scientists now require great amounts of funding, and there is increasing pressure for researchers to make money. Commercialization of research is now a big part of the world we live in. The way forward would be to try to find a balance between the desire for commercialization and the need for good research that is of practical benefit to the public. Since being diagnosed with BRCA2, I have often thought about suing the owners of my gene for all the trouble it has caused me, including out-of-pocket expenses!

We all know we can take every possible precaution in any situation only to be subject to happenstance. We could be hit by a bus, get bitten by a brown snake, die of septicemia from a pinprick wound that was exposed to potting mix. Heck, I heard of a woman once who was hit by a dead duck falling out of the sky while she was changing a flat tire in the middle of nowhere. Chance is a factor that at this point of human evolution we cannot control and we must still allow for.

I have identified one gene mutation in my body and dealt with it according to my best judgment. What about all the other mutant genes I still have in there? What about the other twenty-five thousand genes in the million billion cells in my body? I wonder where it will stop. Will I continue to cut off various bits of my body that potentially may cause me problems in the future? I am still deciding about removing my ovaries, and my doctor suggests the uterus should go too, seeing as I no longer need it. I need to keep in mind that I also have a million billion cells in my body that contain brilliantly healthy genes.

Will we begin to forget that it is a natural process for the human body to die? Human vanity has long led us on the impossible quest for immortality, from expensive beauty creams promising to reverse the aging process to human cryopreservation. Genetic futures could potentially add decades onto our lives, but what about respecting the cycle of life?

We are born to die. The living bit in the middle is the

fun bit, but it is just the bit in the middle. I recognize this more tangibly now that I am a mother. Kaspar is always asking me about life and death, and the more I tease out these concepts with him, the more I understand what my purpose on this earth is. I'm not professing to understand my entire purpose, but part of it, I know, is to move on one day and give others the chance to live.

Kaspar decided that he had a theory about life and death from the age of three. He explained, "We are born as a baby, and then we play, and then we die, and then we come back as a baby and play all over again, and then we die" . . . and so on and so forth. Sounds like a good enough theory for me.

Life has always been a journey of choices, regardless of the advances in technology. The array of choices will just be different. Advancements in humankind's capacity for understanding has always brought with it ethical dilemmas. But just as the industrial age has led us to decimate the very environment we rely on for existence, it will be imperative to find a balance that offers benefits for all of humanity.

21

breast wishes

. . . .

After I returned home from my swap-over surgery, I received a call out of the blue from an old girlfriend of mine, Annie. Not that Annie is old—she is but a few years ahead of me—but our friendship goes back about fifteen years. We had been in a show together called *The Shaugraun* in 1994. It was a rollicking Irish romp; we all had lilting Irish accents, pretty dresses, and long wigs. This show was so much fun it hurt, and Annie and I became great friends. But as it is with most shows, it's hard to keep relationships going outside the environment of the world you have created.

When you meet a cast and create a show, you forge really strong relationships with your fellow actors, becoming like an instant family. You get to know each other in an intense and unnaturally compressed time frame. You also have to find ways to implicitly trust each other because performing is such a team sport. By the end of the show, you feel like you love these people, have known them forever, and will continue to be close to them. Sadly it rarely transpires like that. Time seems to dilute the bonds you created as sure as you move on to a new actor family. Also, actors are itinerants, and it's hard to keep track of people. It took me a long time to learn to let go and move on as one world ended and a new one was ready to be invented.

So Annie and I had not spoken for at least ten years, but she had just been talking to my friend Queenie, who was in the film *Girl Clock* with me. Queenie was telling Annie of my BRCA2 saga, so congratulations must go to the little gene for reuniting Annie and me. Apparently for the last few years, her family too had been unearthing the sinister presence of BRCA2 through their history.

Annie has three sisters. Her younger sister, Amanda, developed breast cancer at thirty-seven years of age. Because she was quite young and her grandmother had died of breast cancer at the age of forty, they tested her for the gene mutation. She was positive.

All of Amanda's sisters—Annie, Caroline, and Kate—decided to be tested, as well as their mother. Only Kate and her mother drew a positive result. I was fascinated to learn that Annie's mother was gene positive and had not gone on to develop breast cancer. I realize there must be people out there with the BRCA2 gene who represent the small percentage of carriers who are not affected by breast cancer, but I had never actually heard of such a person. Every person in my history who was a carrier was unequivocally affected. It was enlightening to think that, with a bit of luck, you could just outsmart the little sucker of a mutant.

Amanda had a mastectomy and chemotherapy and then went on to have a reconstruction. She is forty-one now and considering removal of her ovaries. Kate, on the other hand, was thirty-three and gene positive, and she had not had any breast cancer. She had a young child, and she and her husband knew they wanted another. The gene test seemed to fast-track their baby plans as her doctor advised them to go ahead and have another child, then have the breast removed prophylactically.

Kate had an MRI that showed no tissue changes, so off she went and got pregnant. She told me that when the ultrasound revealed her baby was a boy, she was relieved because the gene mutation is so much riskier for girls. Kate also told me that she encountered some unexpected prejudice when a work colleague questioned her decision to bear another child considering her BRCA2 status.

I would have poked this "Miss Perfect" in the eye, myself; such an attitude implicates you as some sort of criminal who knowingly passes on a faulty gene. Imagine how many gene mutations we are all carrying around; could "Miss Perfect" assure her fetus a perfect genetic code? No one in the world would ever have a child if we all thought like "Miss Perfect." The human race would become extinct, and it would be all her fault.

Eight months after Kate's second son was born, she had a prophylactic mastectomy. She did not keep her skin or nipples. She had a reconstruction and later a nipple reconstruction. Kate's results from her reconstruction have been troublesome, and four surgeries later, she is tired of the soap opera. It is not just the aesthetics of her new breasts—they are still causing her a lot of discomfort. She has what's known as symmastia, in which the area between the breasts pulls away from the sternum and the implants touch. This is also called "kissing implants" or "uniboob." After all the pain she's endured, all she wants is a set of boobs that look vaguely like boobs.

Kate is also considering what to do about her ovaries. She is only thirty-five at present and is very worried about premature menopause. She is hoping that before too long there will be a medical miracle that prevents her from getting ovarian cancer without the sudden and unwelcome arrival of menopause.

My beautiful friend Annie does not have BRCA2 or breast cancer, and I am so glad for her. She did, however, suffer some "survivor guilt." When Amanda was diagnosed with breast cancer, Annie felt completely useless. Unable to take away her sister's pain or help her prognosis in any tangible way, Annie channeled her fears and anxieties into something she could control: the crucible of creativity that transforms adversity into that which is greater than the sum of its parts. She wrote a musical.

Breast Wishes is a beautiful, witty, and funny show about boobs. It journeys through the trials and tribulations of the humble breast. From its budding beginnings, through the battleground of size issues, traversing the slippery slope of sexual titillations, the pain and pleasure of becoming a milk machine, and the deep despair of cancer diagnosis.

Chrissy and I were now officially breast cancer "previvors," and we were dressing up and going out to see a show about . . . you guessed it: BOOBS! We went to the Brisbane opening night, on Annie's invitation. Walking into the theater, I saw a sea of pink; ladies wearing pink feather boas and pink flowers in their hair. The pink breast cancer campaign has been such a success in our country, and we should be proud and confident that the power of pink will see us through to the inevitable discovery of a cure.

There were bras hanging all around the auditorium. I was checking them out, now that I know I am a 12C, imagining what my new breasts would look like in this one and that. I felt very comfortable with how my reconstructed boobs blended in with the veritable feast of mammaries that had turned out for the show.

I felt a certain pride as I walked in, like I was one of the survivors of this dreaded disease. This musical was about the likes of me. I found myself, in the pre-show banter, freely mentioning that I'd had a mastectomy, and I was soaking up the waves of sympathy with a kind of self-satisfaction. My sister, on the other hand, kept complaining that she felt like a fraud, that she was not a survivor, that she didn't belong to any group, that she had slipped through the cracks of pity. I kept telling her that she belonged to the group of "pre-vivors," but that didn't cut the mustard as far as she was concerned.

I know how she feels. It's frustrating when I'm trying to explain to someone what I have actually been through. I say, "I've had a double mastectomy" and then watch as the person realizes with horror that that means the big C: cancer. They say, "Wow, you poor thing," and then follows, "But you're all right now?" I cringe as I am forced to clarify: "Yes. You see, I didn't actually have breast cancer." And then compassion turns to confusion, and I can feel suspicion fill the space between. I really would rather not have to go into the full justification of removing my seemingly healthy breasts because I expose myself to subjective and mostly ill-informed opinions. It would be easier to say I am a breast cancer survivor, but I can't.

The audience was delighted with the show—men and women alike. They laughed as they identified with the myriad of mammary issues presented through songs and scenes. I love the theater. It brings hundreds of strangers together to sit in the dark and share a visceral human experience. It's not like the movies because there is an exchange of energy between the actor and the audience in live theater. And it is a unique, transient experience; what passes between the actors and the audience will never happen again.

In the show, they talked of the history of the brassiere, mentioning when, in 1889, Herminie Cadolle of France first emancipated women from corsetry. The physical and moral constraints of the corset had too long perpetuated the myth that women were the weaker sex. There was a scene in which a well-endowed woman complained of her breasts always engaging in conversation with the opposite sex without her permission. There was the breastfeeding mother's scene, in which one mother suffered the humiliation of bringing out the "formula of failure" in public as she lost the battle to breastfeed.

Breast Wishes also touched on the male experience of breasts. The fact that they were born to look, compulsively, and can't help it. The terror of having a spouse who has to go through the lonely pain of mastectomy and chemotherapy no matter how much support he tries to give her.

In the end, the show turns to the experience of breast cancer for one of the characters. It is sensitive and intelligent in the way it deals with the ultimate downfall of one woman's breasts. I can't help but see breast cancer as a betrayal. We have these mounds that we carry around on our fronts that overshadow or undermine almost everything we do. They suckle and ensure the survival of subsequent generations, and then they betray us by trying to kill us. Why our breasts? Why do they have to be so potentially deadly? It's like a bad joke, a crappy design fault.

Luckily for me, *Breast Wishes* was a coolant for my overheating emotions. The show eventually persuaded me to "be kind to my breasts." It made me realize I had been very angry with the injustice of it all. Not just what had happened to me but the struggle all women have had to face: my mother, Elsie, Maude, Chrissy, Sue, and Kate. But I do; I have to be kind to my breasts in spite of it all—they are just trying to survive. We are trying to survive together.

After the show, there were a few speeches. I learned that Annie and her producers arranged for the National Breast Cancer Foundation to be the recipient of royalties from Breast Wishes. So Annie really did make a tangible difference, and she will be partly responsible for finding a cure for breast cancer. A representative of the National Breast Cancer Foundation spoke after the show, and she really brought us all to tears. I had come so far on this trail and had hardly shed a tear. This is partly a Neave trait—we drown everything in laughter instead of tears. Sometimes you feel that if you were to start you may never stop, but it's a risk you have to take, I guess.

What made me cry was comprehending that in Australia breast cancer is the most invasive cancer among women. Each year in Australia, around 12,000 women are diagnosed with the disease and around 2,600 women die from it. These are the statistics, and I have been wading in statistics on breast cancer for years now. But they are not just numbers; they are lives. They are someone's daughter, sister, mother, aunt, grandmother.

I cried for the people who this disease leaves behind. I kind of escaped the full force of grief because I did not lose my mother and Maude and Elsie died before I was born. But my heart went out to those people who are truly grieving because of breast cancer. And my tears fell because I thought of Kaspar and the grief I hope that I have spared him.

It was wonderful to see Annie again after all these years. We hugged, we laughed, she felt my boobs! I proudly introduced my sister around too. Normally at opening nights my sister feels a bit out of place and overwhelmed; overwhelmed by the arrogance of actors, that is. She doesn't understand that we're not necessarily arrogant, but mostly just overwhelmed ourselves when we come out and meet our audience face-to-face. We have exposed ourselves up there on the stage and now have to come out and talk to total strangers as ourselves, and this makes us feel slightly inadequate. Not that I have ever convinced her of that. We are just rude and stuck-up and only like to talk about ourselves, apparently. But she was not out of place that night; she had a right to be there— she'd had a mastectomy. I think it was good for us both.

epilogue

I see Dr. D for my post-op check-up, exactly one year after my mastectomy, to check on the success of his back boob wrangling. He seems happy enough with his work. So am I, but I tell him I don't ever wish to see him again. I say to him that it's over—our relationship, it's over. I tell him that I realize that I was not the only one. I tell him that I know there are other women in the waiting room that have come to see him and that he will touch their breasts just as he is touching mine now. I tell him it has been rich and real but I don't ever want to see his shiny blue eyes again. Well, not for a while. We need some space. Perhaps in the future when my boobs need replacing and I want an upgrade to DD because I'm having a midlife crisis.

I really hope I can stop myself from doing the washing or vacuuming for the next three weeks. I just don't want to bust these stitches again. But it's so hard to not attend to my house in this way. Kaspar's sheets need changing and so do mine, and I am loath to call my sister to come over after work and do my housework. Sam has been a wonderful "Sadie the cleaning lady" for the last week but is now on tour. I don't want to have another operation, so I will make myself live in squalor for as long as I can possibly stand it. Dr. D has stitched my boob up beautifully, and if they stay this way, I can honestly say that they look like a very nice set of breasts, even if they don't feel that way.

Back home, I determine to love my breasts as they are now or however they will be. I have interfered enough, and now I shall just let them be. I have a feeling that the sensations are returning slightly. The other day I was playing with Kaspar. He was on my back, and I was trying to throw him off, which I did eventually, but he grabbed onto my right breast to try to save himself from falling. He fell nonetheless, but his little fingernails dug in until the last, and I actually felt it! I felt it for the next three days. It was not the normal sensation of someone ripping your skin with their fingernails, but it was something. I am led to believe that some sensation can be restored as nerves are reformed. I think this may help me to feel like these breasts are really part of me.

Kaspar is five, and I'm sure he'll forget that Mummy ever had an operation on her boobies, but when he is old enough, I guess I will tell him that he has a 50 percent chance of inheriting this gene. He will have to decide for himself what he will do about it when it comes time for him to procreate.

Chrissy's son David also will have to make a choice to test or not to test when he is considering a family. He already knows his mother has the gene, so he cannot ignore the fact that it is in his family; it is a difficult choice for him either way.

Denny apparently is going to have the gene test as soon as he can get around to it—he's a busy boy. His partner Sharon is on his case to have it because he is of an age where prostate cancer becomes an issue for men, and his BRCA2 status will increase his risk in this area.

Chrissy, Mum, and I have dodged the curve ball so far; but it does feel like just that—we have only dodged it. Chrissy has been back to Dr. D, concerned about some pain and swelling that occurs occasionally: he really wants to operate again and remove some more tissue that he is worried about. BRCA2 still has our family firmly in its sights for future generations. If Denny is negative, David is negative, John is negative, Jack is negative, and Kaspar is negative, then we will have bred out the BRCA2 gene in our lineage, no problem.

Foxtel Biography and the national broadcaster ABC purchased our documentary. This is a great outcome because it means that a large part of the population will gain a little more awareness on this issue. It is a bit of a coup, really, seeing as my brother had never made a documentary before. Foxtel Bio continues to run the documentary, and we are humbled and honored to share this space with stories of such amazing strength and power. The ABC views hundreds of documentaries each week and purchases only a fraction of these. There is a satisfaction for all of us that our story will hopefully provide more women and families with information on what BRCA2 means.

My next job is taking *The Age I'm In* on an international tour. We are heading to Dublin, Montreal, and Seoul. So my new breasts will get to see the world. You never know, they may even meet someone of the opposite sex who is attracted to them. I'm not sure how I will cope with this, to be honest. I will just have to cross that bridge if I ever come to it. But for now there is just dry, dry land!

I have fought the BRCA2 gene—my sister and mother have also gone rounds, but I'm not sure any of us have won. My little sister Loo Loo, who thought she had time on her side being only thirty years old, has just found a lump in her breast. She has had a mammogram and an ultrasound, and they want to do a biopsy. It's relentless, this gene; terrorizing our family without remorse. We will all hold our breath until her results, and if all is good, we'll try to breathe easy—until the next time.

about *the* author

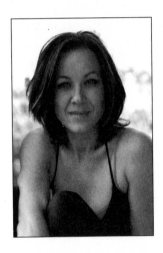

Veronica Neave grew up in Australia as an army brat, moving every few years to a new post. She attended drama classes from the age of five, ultimately leading to a degree in "the arts" and a reputation as a highly respected theater actor, acclaimed nationally and internationally. With a career stretching over twenty years, she has appeared in over fifty stage productions within Australia, from Shakespeare and Tennessee Williams to writing and appearing in various shows with Kate Champion's Force Majeure. She has also appeared in a number of TV series. In 2008, she completed filming as the lead in an Australian film, *Girl Clock*. Known for her versatility in the Arts industry, she is a performer, writer, teacher, and director.

Veronica continues to perform in theater in Australia and abroad. Although she has written for theater for many years, this is her first book.

DATE DUE

The Library Store #47-0152